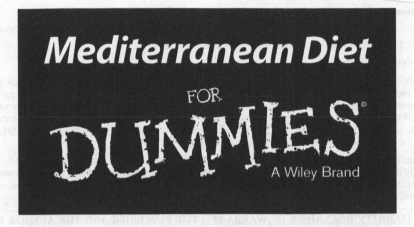

Mediterranean Diet

FOR

DUMMIES

A Wiley Brand

by Rachel Berman, RD, CD/N

Mediterranean Diet For Dummies®

Published by: **John Wiley & Sons, Inc.,** 111 River Street, Hoboken, NJ 07030-5774, www.wiley.com

Copyright © 2013 by John Wiley & Sons, Inc., Hoboken, New Jersey

Published simultaneously in Canada

No part of this publication may be reproduced, stored in a retrieval system or transmitted in any form or by any means, electronic, mechanical, photocopying, recording, scanning or otherwise, except as permitted under Sections 107 or 108 of the 1976 United States Copyright Act, without the prior written permission of the Publisher. Requests to the Publisher for permission should be addressed to the Permissions Department, John Wiley & Sons, Inc., 111 River Street, Hoboken, NJ 07030, (201) 748-6011, fax (201) 748-6008, or online at http://www.wiley.com/go/permissions.

Trademarks: Wiley, For Dummies, the Dummies Man logo, Dummies.com, Making Everything Easier, and related trade dress are trademarks or registered trademarks of John Wiley & Sons, Inc., and may not be used without written permission. All other trademarks are the property of their respective owners. John Wiley & Sons, Inc., is not associated with any product or vendor mentioned in this book.

For general information on our other products and services, please contact our Customer Care Department within the U.S. at 877-762-2974, outside the U.S. at 317-572-3993, or fax 317-572-4002. For technical support, please visit www.wiley.com/techsupport.

Wiley publishes in a variety of print and electronic formats and by print-on-demand. Some material included with standard print versions of this book may not be included in e-books or in print-on-demand. If this book refers to media such as a CD or DVD that is not included in the version you purchased, you may download this material at http://booksupport.wiley.com. For more information about Wiley products, visit www.wiley.com.

Library of Congress Control Number: 2013942768

ISBN 978-1-118-71525-3 (pbk); ISBN 978-1-118-71530-7 (ebk); ISBN 978-1-118-71533-8 (ebk); ISBN 978-1-118-71534-5 (ebk)

Manufactured in the United States of America

SKY10051645_072123

Contents at a Glance

Recipes at a Glance

Table of Contents

Introduction

●●●

*O*n the television, on radio, and in newspapers and magazines (both print and online), we're bombarded with ads for diets that purport to melt away the unwanted pounds, books touting "proven" diet weight loss plans, and rumor mill diets that usually involve some whacky dietary requirement, like eating only peanut butter and pickles for three days straight or some other such nonsense.

Here's a not-too-well-hidden secret: *These diets things don't work.* At least not in terms of losing weight and not in terms of improving health. A diet that *does* work is the Mediterranean diet.

What makes this diet different? It's not really a diet, at least not the "give up all the good stuff you love and live on celery sticks and sugar-free popsicles" variety. Instead, it's a way of eating and living that celebrates good food, connections to family and friends, stress management, and work and play. In other words, it's a lifestyle that embraces all that life has to offer.

What's truly amazing, however, is that this lifestyle isn't some fad: It's existed in the Mediterranean region for years, where folks have been so healthy — living longer and avoiding health conditions that have plagued people in other parts of the world — that researchers took notice. Over decades of study and numerous research projects, they demonstrated a direct link between the diet and beneficial health outcomes.

About This Book

With all the information floating around out there about the Mediterranean diet, you've probably heard dribs and drabs about the good things it does (reduces the risk of diabetes, for example) and how it does it (it involves using a lot of olive oil or nuts, for instance). You may even have heard inaccurate information (you can't eat red meat anymore).

This book puts all the key information in one place, describing the conditions that the diet has been shown to positively influence, identifying the key food groups that make up the Mediterranean diet food pyramid, outlining the diet's key principles, and explaining how to incorporate these principles into your own life.

It's quite a bit of information, and to help you find what you're looking for, we've divided the discussions into parts, each focusing on a particular topic. One part, for example, is devoted to the health conditions and another to the key foods in the diet. This organization lets you go directly to the information that most interests you. And for those discussion that aren't vital to your understanding of the Mediterranean diet, we identify them as skippable by putting them in a shaded box or marking them with a special icon.

Within this book, you may also note that some web addresses break across two lines of text. If you're reading this book in print and want to visit one of these web pages, simply key in the web address exactly as it's noted in the text, pretending as though the line break doesn't exist. If you're reading this as an e-book, you've got it easy — just click the web address to be taken directly to the web page.

And because this book includes a chapter with recipes, we've established a few conventions to avoid any confusion:

- ✔ All eggs are large.
- ✔ All milk is low-fat unless otherwise specified.
- ✔ All pepper is freshly ground black pepper unless otherwise specified.
- ✔ All salt is kosher.
- ✔ All temperatures are Fahrenheit (see the appendix to convert Fahrenheit temperatures to Celsius).
- ✔ All lemon and lime juice is freshly squeezed.
- ✔ All flour is all-purpose white flour unless otherwise noted.
- ○ This little tomato icon highlights the recipes in this book that don't include meat or meat products.

Foolish Assumptions

In writing this book, we made some assumptions about you:

- ✔ You love food that is both delicious and healthy and have heard that a Mediterranean-based diet offers both.
- ✔ You want to reduce your risk of developing various diseases or, if you have already developed chronic conditions (like high blood pressure or diabetes), you want to mitigate the severity of the symptoms.

✔ You want to know more about the health claims made about the Mediterranean diet.

✔ You're interested in transitioning a protein-and-starch–based diet to a plant-based diet.

✔ You're game for any diet that lets you consume fats and nuts without guilt.

Icons Used in This Book

To help you find certain kinds of information easily, this book uses the following icons:

This icon appears beside shortcuts and recommendations that can save you time, money, or frustration.

This icon highlights key principle or fundamental points that you need to remember.

If something poses a danger — to your health, your safety, or your wallet — you'll see this icon beside it.

Some of the information in this book is just fun or interesting, but not vital to your being able to incorporate the Mediterranean diet into your life. When you see this icon, feel free to move on past without reading.

You can find a lot of good information online at www.dummies.com/extras/ mediterraneandiet. This icon points the way.

Beyond the Book

In addition to the material in the print or e-book you're reading right now, this product also comes with some goodies you can access on the web. Check out the free Cheat Sheet at www.dummies.com/cheatsheet/ mediterraneandiet for information on how to use olive oil in your cooking, a quick guide to serving sizes, and what wines to pair with what foods.

Head to www.dummies.com/extras/mediterraneandiet to find pointers on how to quit smoking, the nutritional benefits of several foods highlighted in the Mediterranean diet, how to increase you activity level simply by walking more, and advice on using olive oil in your cooking.

Where to Go from Here

One of the nice things about this book is that it's designed to be a reference. You can go to any topic and find all the information you need right there. You don't need to start at the beginning and read through to the end.

If you already know the kind of information you're looking for, simply go to the index at the back of the book or the table of contents at the front, and scan through until you find what you're looking for. Alternatively, you can simply flip through the pages to see what strikes your fancy and begin reading there.

Of course, if you don't know where to begin, the beginning is always a good place to start. For those of you who want to jump right in, why not try out the recipe chapter — head directly to Chapter 16. If you want to know about a particular health condition, head to Part II. Wherever you go, you're bound to find interesting and illuminating information.

In Italy, they say, "Buon appetito!" In Spain, "¡Que aproveche!" In Greece, "Kalí óreksi!" But the phrase in Morocco — "Bil-hanā' wa ash-shifā'" — best epitomizes the Mediterranean diet:

"May you have your meal with gladness and good health."

Part I

Getting Started with the Mediterranean Diet

getting started with the Mediterranean Diet

Visit www.dummies.com for great Dummies content online.

In this part . . .

- ✔ Get up to speed on the principles of the Mediterranean diet, like eating healthy fats, increasing the amount of fruits and vegetables, opting for lean protein sources rather than fatty ones, and devoting time to relaxation and fun.

- ✔ Examine how the dietary and lifestyle components of the Mediterranean diet can improve heart health, reduce cancer risk, prevent or mitigate the problems associated with diabetes, and help you maintain a healthy weight.

Chapter 1

A Guided Tour through the Mediterranean Diet

In This Chapter

▶ Discovering the key components of the Mediterranean diet

▶ Recognizing key differences between the Mediterranean diet and a traditional Western diet

▶ Taking a look at the health benefits

The Mediterranean diet is a way of life — one where you eat lots of fresh food and slow down. More technically, the Mediterranean diet is a modern set of guidelines inspired by traditional diet patterns of southern Italy, the Greek island of Crete, and other parts of Greece. The lifestyle was first researched in the 1960s, and in 2010, the United Nations Educational, Scientific and Cultural Organization (UNESCO) officially recognized this diet pattern to be part of the cultural heritage of Italy, Greece, Spain, and Morocco. A more rural lifestyle is a common thread among all these regions.

This chapter gives you an overview of the Mediterranean diet, explaining what it is, what it includes, and how it's more than just a food plan; it's also a way to embrace and enjoy life.

Introducing the Mediterranean Diet

The Mediterranean Sea, connected to the Atlantic Ocean by the thin (14-mile wide) Strait of Gibraltar in the west and to the Sea of Marmara and the Black Sea by the Dardanelles and the Bosporus in the east, has long played an important role in the civilizations that border it. Surrounded by the coastlines of 21 countries — Algeria, Croatia, Cyprus, Egypt, France, Greece, Italy, Libya, Malta, Montenegro, and Spain to name just a few — it has been an important route for merchants and travelers and a primary source of food for the civilizations that sprang up around it. The climate in the Mediterranean region — hot and dry in the summer and mild and rainy in the winter — lends itself to crops like olives, figs, and grapes; and the rocky, coastal terrain is more suitable for sheep, goats, and chicken than that staple of traditional western diets: beef. The nearby sea provides an abundance and variety of seafood.

This region has long fascinated and inspired the Western world in terms of governance, philosophy, science, mathematics, art, architecture, and more. Now, studies that draw direct links between what is called the Mediterranean diet and reduced risks for heart disease, reduced incidence of cancer and cancer deaths, and reduced incidence of Parkinson's and Alzheimer's diseases have given people another reason to embrace the Mediterranean.

The Mediterranean diet relies on fruits and vegetables, lean protein sources, and healthy fats — hallmarks of all healthy diets. So you may be wondering what makes this diet different. Here's a quick overview of the Mediterranean diet and its effects; the next sections provide a fuller introductions to these concepts:

- ✔ **The recommended proportions:** If you look at the Mediterranean food pyramid (see Figure 1-1), you can see a couple of interesting things, the first of which is that the food groups you may be accustomed to (dairy, meats and other proteins, fruits, and vegetables) are regrouped. Specifically, all the plant-based foods — fruits, vegetables, and foods (like grains, legumes, nuts, olives, olive oil, herbs, and spices) that come from plants — are all in one group, and the proteins are divided into no less than three categories, with chicken grouped with dairy products, and red meat stuck at the top with sweets! This division is a key reason why the Mediterranean diet is so healthful: it includes a specific balance of foods that are high in vitamins, minerals, and antioxidants and contain the optimum balance of fatty acids.

- ✔ **The holistic nature of the diet:** The second thing you may notice about the food pyramid is that its foundation isn't a food group. It's a call to live a physically active life and to enjoy meals with others.

The Mediterranean Food Guide Pyramid is based on the dietary traditions of the Greek island of Crete, other parts of Greece, and southern Italy around 1960, when chronic diseases such as heart disease and cancer were low. As Figure 1-1 shows, the focus is on eating a diet rich in vegetables, fruits, whole grains, legumes, and seafood; eating less meat; and choosing healthy fats such as olive oil. Note also the importance of fun activities, time shared with family and friends, and a passion for life.

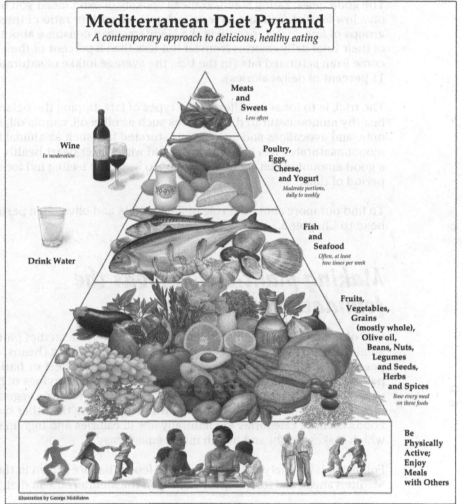

Mediterranean Diet Pyramid
A contemporary approach to delicious, healthy eating

Meats and Sweets
Less often

Wine
In moderation

Poultry, Eggs, Cheese, and Yogurt
Moderate portions, daily to weekly

Drink Water

Fish and Seafood
Often, at least two times per week

Fruits, Vegetables, Grains (mostly whole), Olive oil, Beans, Nuts, Legumes and Seeds, Herbs and Spices
Base every meal on these foods

Be Physically Active; Enjoy Meals with Others

Illustration by George Middleton

© 2009 Oldways Preservation & Exchange Trust," www.oldwayspt.org

Figure 1-1: The Mediterranean Food Guide Pyramid.

Cooking with healthy fats

Although Mediterranean residents don't consume a low-fat diet, their dietary pattern is considered heart-healthy. How can that be? Because not all fats are created equal. People in the Mediterranean consume more of the healthier types of fats (monounsaturated fats and polyunsaturated omega-3 fatty acids) and less of the omega-6 polyunsaturated fatty acids and saturated fats other cultures tend to overload on.

The good news: Eating Mediterranean cooking doesn't mean you have to go on a low-fat diet. You just have to maintain a healthier ratio of these different groups of fats. In fact, people in the Mediterranean consume about 35 percent of their total daily calories from fat but less than 8 percent of their calories come from saturated fats (in the U.S., the average intake of saturated fats is 11 percent of daily calories).

The trick is to focus on different the types of fats, tipping the balance toward healthy monounsaturated fat sources such as olive oil, canola oil, olives, nuts, and avocadoes and away from saturated fats such as animal fats. Using monounsaturated fats is often associated with better heart health. Eating a good amount of dietary fat also helps to keep you feeling full for a longer period of time.

To find out more about the role of healthy fats and olive oil in particular, head to Chapter 8.

Making plant-based foods the foundation of every meal

One of the most important concepts of the Mediterranean diet pattern is consuming lots of plant foods such as fruits, veggies, legumes (beans, lentils, and peas, for example), and whole grains, such as bulgur wheat or barley. In fact, people in the Mediterranean commonly eat five to ten servings of fruits and vegetables each day, which often means having two to three vegetable servings with each meal. The legume and whole grains are the other daily staples. Foods in these categories are naturally low in calories and high in nutrients, which makes weight and health management easy.

Following is a variety of the plant-based foods that are grown in the Mediterranean and feature prominently in the Mediterranean diet:

- **Legumes:** Chickpeas, lentils, peas
- **Fruits:** Olives, mandarin oranges, figs, grapes, lemons, persimmons, pomegranates
- **Grains:** Barley, corn, rice, wheat
- **Nuts:** Almonds, hazelnuts, pine nuts, walnuts
- **Vegetables:** Asparagus, broccoli, cabbage, green beans, garlic, onions, eggplant, tomatoes, broccoli rabe, artichokes

Chapters 9 through 11 feature the details of the benefits of all these plant-based foods.

Eating seafood weekly

Seafood is a weekly staple in the Mediterranean diet, and with good reason. First, it's a local product. The least expensive seafood in the Mediterranean region includes sardines, anchovies, mackerel, squid, and octopus. Mid-priced fish and shellfish include tuna, trout, clams, and mussels. For a pricey, special occasion meal, options include lobster and red mullet.

During the 1960s, before the area was over-fished, a variety of seafood was available in the Mediterranean. Unfortunately, fish stocks today are significantly low due to overfishing, and many important species, such as tuna, are threatened.

Second, seafood is a great source of those coveted omega-3 fatty acids. You can add seafood to a few weekly meals and reap the same benefits. If you live near a coast, you have a great opportunity to find fresh fish in your local stores and restaurants. If you're landlocked, don't discount lakes and rivers for fresh fish.

Check out http://www.montereybayaquarium.org/cr/seafoodwatch. aspx for a list of recommended fish in your region. This guide is a great tool to help you choose local fish with low contaminants and also to protect against overfishing. Don't like fish? You can get omega-3 fatty acids in other ways, such as with fish oil supplements or by eating lots of fresh herbs, walnuts, and flaxseeds.

Limiting your consumption of red meat

Many people automatically consider protein foods such as beef, poultry, pork, and fish as an entree. But in the Mediterranean, beef is only served once or twice a month rather than several times a week, as it is in many U.S. kitchens. And when it does hit the table, it's usually as a small (2- to 3-ounce) side dish rather than an 8-plus-ounce entree. This habit helps ensure a reasonable intake of saturated fats and omega-6 fatty acids. (See the earlier section "Cooking with healthy fats" for info on why balancing fat intake is important.)

Red meat used to be a luxury item in rural parts of the Mediterranean, so folks there ate it less frequently. Even though it's now more accessible to the average Joe, the serving limits have stuck over the years.

Before you panic, keep in mind that the Mediterranean diet doesn't require that you eliminate all red meat. The goal is simply to eat less animal protein and more plant-based protein. Fortunately, you can easily replace a portion of your traditional meat serving with lentils or beans to add plant-based protein to your meals. For example, instead of having an 8-ounce steak, you may choose to have a 3- or 4-ounce portion but also have a lentil salad or sprinkle some nuts on a salad. This strategy also helps you add more vegetable servings to help fill the plate.

Who knows? You may even discover that you don't miss the meat. Because of their use of spices and herbs, many Mediterranean recipes featuring beef, for example, are so full of flavor that a small serving becomes more satisfying.

You can find what you need to know about both seafood and animal protein sources in Chapter 12.

Using dairy in moderation

You may think of the Mediterranean as a cheese-eater's heaven, but the truth is that people in the Mediterranean areas from which this diet comes don't consume an abundance of cheese. Dairy is consumed on a daily basis in the Mediterranean diet, and cheese (along with yogurt) is a common source of calcium; however, moderation is the key.

Incorporate two to three servings of dairy products daily. One serving may include an 8-ounce glass of milk, 8 ounces of yogurt, or 1 ounce of cheese. Stick with the low-fat versions of milk and yogurt to help lower your saturated fat intake; because you're eating so little of it, you can go with regular cheese if you want.

Enhancing flavor with herbs and spices

Fresh herbs and spices not only add tremendous flavor to food but also have many hidden health benefits. Oregano and basil in your spaghetti sauce, for example, do more than provide a distinct Italian flavor; those herbs are also plants, which means they have all sorts of health benefits that can make a big impact on your overall health. Simple seasonings such as ginger and oregano contain *phytochemicals,* which are natural health-promoting substances that have been found to protect against conditions such as cancer and heart disease.

You may be surprised to hear that herbs and spices are also loaded with healthy omega-3 fatty acids, which help decrease inflammation in the body. Check out some of the specific health benefits of commonly used herbs and spices:

✔ Basil is shown to have anti-inflammatory effects and may be useful for people with chronic inflammation, such as arthritis or inflammatory bowel disease. Basil also protects against bacteria and is an excellent source of vitamin A, which helps reduce damage to the body from free radicals.

✔ Cinnamon helps people better control their blood sugars because it slows digestion and therefore the rise of blood sugar — not to mention that it's a wonderful flavor for baking or in a cup of tea!

✔ Oregano is a nutrient-dense spice containing fiber, iron, manganese, calcium, vitamin C, vitamin A, and omega-3 fatty acids. It's shown to have antibacterial and antioxidant properties.

✔ Parsley is a rich source of the antioxidants vitamin A and vitamin C, providing protection from heart disease and cancer. (And you thought eating your parsley garnish was silly.)

✔ Turmeric acts as a powerful anti-inflammatory and antioxidant, helping protect against arthritis, heart disease, and certain cancers.

Other herbs and spices common to Mediterranean cooking include rosemary, sage, dill, thyme, mint, and fennel.

If you already use ample herbs and spices in your own cooking, you're on the right track. If not, try to discover new flavors and ways to add more of these plants into your diet. Chapter 17 lists ten must-have spices to add to your repertoire.

Drinking wine with your meals

Drinking a glass of wine with dinner is certainly a common practice in the Mediterranean regions. Red wine has special nutrients that are shown to be heart-healthy; however, moderation is important. Enjoying some red wine a couple times a week is certainly a good plan for heart health, although you want to check with your doctor to ensure it's okay for you. Check out Chapter 13 for specifics on the benefits of red wine.

Embracing life

Historically, the people in the rural Mediterranean got plenty of daily activity through work, getting where they needed to go on foot, and having fun. Although you may rely heavily on your car and think the Mediterranean lifestyle isn't realistic for you, you can still find ways to incorporate both aerobic exercise (which gets your heart rate up) and strength-training exercises regularly.

Walking encompasses both aerobic and strength training and helps relieve stress. If you live close to markets or restaurants, challenge yourself to walk to them rather than drive, or simply focus on taking a walk each day to unwind.

Community spirit is a large part of the Mediterranean culture and is something that's disappearing in American culture. Getting together on a regular basis with friends and family is an important priority for providing a sense of strong community and fun. The fun and laughter that come with friendly get-togethers are vital for stress management. Without these little joyful experiences, stress can tip to an unhealthy balance.

To put this strategy into practice, invite some of your close family and friends over each week, perhaps for dinner. It can be as casual as you like. The important thing is to add this type of fun and enjoyment to your life more often.

The Mediterranean coast is full of sunshine, good food, and beautiful surroundings, so the people who live there naturally tend to have a strong passion for life, family, friends, nature, and food. Choosing to have a strong passion and love of life is associated with more happiness and fulfillment and less stress. So what are you passionate about? Perhaps you love the arts, or maybe nature is your thing. Whatever your passions are, make sure to find a way to make them a regular part of your life.

Chapter 14 describes the Mediterranean lifestyle and offers suggestions on how you can incorporate those qualities into your own life.

Getting Started

The things that differentiate the eating habits of people living on the Mediterranean coast and other cultures are actually quite subtle. These small differences include eating smaller portion sizes and regulating how often certain foods are consumed. The changes may be small, but they make a significant difference for weight management, health, and well-being. You may have trouble believing that such small shifts can really make that big an impact, but they really do.

This section dives into meal planning to show you some small changes based on the Mediterranean lifestyle that have big effects on the amounts of calories and nutrients you consume. You can also find some valuable lifestyle ideas to get you into the Mediterranean spirit.

Identifying the flavors of the Mediterranean coast

As noted previously, 21 countries have coastlines that border the Mediterranean Sea. Having a decent understanding of these countries and their cooking styles can help you have a better appreciation for this way of life.

Table 1-1 lists some of the countries in the Mediterranean that are part of this lifestyle and the associated flavors and cooking styles commonly used in those areas.

Table 1-1	Common Mediterranean Flavors by Region	
Region	*Commonly Used Ingredients*	*Overall Cuisine Flavor*
Southern Italy	Anchovies, balsamic vinegar, basil, bay leaf, capers, garlic, mozzarella cheese, olive oil, oregano, parsley, peppers, pine nuts, mushrooms, prosciutto, rosemary, sage, thyme, tomatoes	Italian food is rich and savory, with strongly flavored ingredients. Look for tomato-based sauces and even an occasional kick of spicy heat.
Greece	Basil, cucumbers, dill, fennel, feta cheese, garlic, honey, lemon, mint, olive oil, oregano, yogurt	Greek cooking runs the gamut from tangy with citrus accents to savory. Ingredients such as feta cheese add a strong, bold flavor, while yogurt helps provide a creamy texture and soft flavor.
Morocco	Cinnamon, cumin, dried fruits, ginger, lemon, mint, paprika, parsley, pepper, saffron, turmeric	Moroccan cooking uses exotic flavors that encompass both sweet and savory, often in one dish. The food has strong flavors but isn't necessarily spicy.
Spain	Almonds, anchovies, cheeses (from goats, cows, and sheep), garlic, ham, honey, olive oil, onions, oregano, nuts, paprika, rosemary, saffron, thyme	Regardless of what part of Spain you're in, you can always count on garlic and olive oil setting the stage for a flavorful dish. Spanish dishes are often inspired by Arabic and Roman cuisine with emphasis on fresh seafood. You often find combinations of savory and sweet flavors, such as a seafood stew using sweet paprika.

Although you may see some of the same ingredients in many recipes, the flavors used in different countries or regions create entirely different dishes. If you've eaten both Italian and Greek meatballs, for example, you know that the two varieties sure don't taste the same.

Grasping the importance of meal planning

Meal planning provides you a road map for the week of what you're going to eat, when you'll prepare those meals, and what foods you need to have handy in your kitchen to do so. By taking the steps to do some planning, changing to a Mediterranean diet is much easier and less stressful.

Meal planning on some level is important for several reasons:

- ✔ It ensures that you're efficient with your time and have everything you need on hand from the grocery store and markets. This preparedness also helps keep you on track with your Mediterranean lifestyle because you always have the fixings for fresh meals at your fingertips.

- ✔ It makes cooking easier during the week because you already know what you're making instead of trying to think of what you can cook with the chicken and cauliflower you bought.

- ✔ It saves you money by decreasing food waste. Do you ever buy broccoli and then wonder what to do with it as it starts yellowing in your refrigerator? Waste.

If you have a pit in your stomach right now and are ready to skip this section, hold on! Meal planning needs to (and can) work into your lifestyle. Here are a few different approaches; hopefully, you find one that works for you:

- ✔ **The detailed meal plan:** This plan is for those who love details and planning. Sit down and write out a plan for breakfast, lunch, and dinner for each day of the week. (You may want to include snacks as well.) You can make each day's foods interchangeable, but this planning method at least makes sure you have a plan and can go on your way this week with everything organized.

- ✔ **The rotating two-week meal plan:** If you like details and convenience, this setup is perfect for you. Spend some time making up a two-week meal plan, complete with shopping list, and you've done all the work you need. You still get plenty of variety with a two-week meal plan, but you may need to change it up every couple of months to make seasonal menus.

✓ **The fast meal plan:** If you don't want to waste time on making a meal plan for each and every meal for the week, think about your habits and plan accordingly. For example, if you regularly eat a few different items for breakfast and usually eat leftovers or sandwiches and fruit for lunch, you can focus planning dinners and the few staples you need for the other meals. And if you typically use leftovers for other meals, making a menu plan for four to five nights a week will work out just fine.

✓ **The super-fast meal plan:** Perhaps you need something even speedier than the fast menu plan. Instead of planning four or five dinners a week, focus on two to three and plan some convenience meals, such as entree salads you can throw together or canned or homemade frozen soups.

Head to Chapter 15 for more ways to make incorporating the Mediterranean diet into a busy life easier.

Changing the way you fill your plate

Folks on the Mediterranean coast eat many of the same foods that people elsewhere do; they just eat smaller portions and incorporate plenty of vegetables. For example, they may eat pizza, but they eat less pizza; go easy on the sauce, cheese, and other toppings; and add a salad and possibly other side vegetables. This section highlights some of the Mediterranean eating habits you can adopt when you're meal planning. These small changes make all the difference in health and flavor.

When you think of a Mediterranean lifestyle and dietary patterns, the focus is on the traditional habits seen at least 50 years ago in the regions noted in this chapter. If you visited northern Italy in a recent trip, you may not have experienced any of the dietary patterns promoted in this book — and no, that huge portion of butter-laden pasta you had doesn't qualify for this diet.

Focusing on plant-based foods

As noted earlier, the Mediterranean climate makes for abundant amounts of fresh fruits and vegetables, and people from the region use what they have on hand. As a result, they eat a lot of plant-based foods (five to ten daily servings of fruits and vegetables) and depend less on prepackaged convenience foods. A typical American diet, on the other hand, includes about three servings of fruits and vegetables a day on average, and prepackaged foods are the go-to items for many meals.

Getting the five to ten fruits and vegetables servings a day is easier when you consider that beans and lentils commonly take the place of smaller meat portion. (See the upcoming section "Finding the right balance with protein" for information on changing your protein mindset.)

Consuming whole grains rather than processed grains

Incorporating whole grains into your daily meal plans provides a great source of complex carbohydrates, fiber, vitamins, and minerals; it also adds flavor and texture to your meals. The trick is to use grains as a smaller side dish to avoid eating too many calories and increasing your blood sugar with too many carbohydrates. Use one-half to one cup of grains with your meals to stay on the healthy side of the fence.

Although people on the Mediterranean coast frequently use pasta, they also consume many other grains, such as bulgur wheat, barley, and cornmeal. Chapter 11 tells you everything you need to know about grains, and Chapter 14 offers cooking tips that make including grains in your meals easy.

Finding the right balance with protein

As we explain earlier, meat is typically a side dish in the Mediterranean diet; when meat does serve as the main dish, it's in a smaller portion size than you're probably used to. Thinking of meat as anything but an entree may be difficult. If you're a meat lover, you may be just about ready to put this book on the shelf because you think you have to give up your favorite foods. Wait! You don't have to become vegetarian to live a Mediterranean lifestyle.

Incorporating this lifestyle is more about eating less and adding more variety to your plate than about depriving yourself completely. The goal isn't to abandon animal protein but simply to eat less of it and more of plant-based protein.

If you feel like this lifestyle isn't for you, consider going halfway. Eating your normal portions of meat two to three days a week and going a more Mediterranean route on the other days may work better for you. If you aren't willing to give up your regular portion of steak, look for other places in the meal where you can incorporate Mediterranean concepts. Start with what you're comfortable with; even a partial change in your habits can make a big difference in your overall health.

Enjoying the Health Benefits Linked to the Mediterranean Diet

The Mediterranean diet has long been touted for providing health benefits, such as reducing coronary artery disease and decreasing the risk of some cancers. Including fresh vegetables and fruits, legumes, and healthy fats into your diet can help improve your health in many ways. Although Chapter 2 provides a more detailed overview of the health benefits and Part II discusses in detail the many chronic conditions that a Mediterranean eating plan can help mitigate, here's a quick rundown of the ways the diet benefits you:

- **Promoting heart health:** Heart disease is the number one cause of death in the United States, even though a few lifestyle changes make most cases of heart disease easily preventable. Studies show that a traditional Mediterranean diet decreases death from coronary artery disease by 9 percent and lowers blood pressure, blood sugar, and triglyceride levels. Chapters 3 and 4 cover heart disease, hypertension, and stroke.

- **Battling diabetes:** The foods in a Mediterranean diet make perfect sense for a person with type 2 diabetes because the food choices lean toward being low-glycemic, which convert to sugar more slowly and therefore tend not to cause blood sugar levels to spike. The portion sizes in the Mediterranean diet can also make a significant difference in keeping total carbohydrate intake during the meal in check. Chapter 5 provides the details on diabetes.

- **Fighting cancer:** Specific staples of the Mediterranean diet have been shown to provide cancer-preventing and cancer-fighting benefits. Head to Chapter 7 for details on that disease.

- **Losing weight:** Obesity is an epidemic in the U.S. and is becoming a major health problem around the world. Therefore, weight loss is an important issue for many people (and perhaps you). If you want to lose some weight, the Mediterranean diet is the way to go. Be forewarned, however: A Mediterranean diet isn't a traditional "diet" or a quick fix. Rather, it's a series of healthy lifestyle choices that can get you to your weight loss goal while you eat delicious, flavorful foods and get out and enjoy life. Chapter 6 has details on the dangers associated with being overweight and how the Mediterranean diet can help.

- **Aging gracefully:** A Mediterranean lifestyle can help you feel and look your best. A diet high in nutrients, moderate activity, and lots of laughter with friends lets you enjoy the benefits of health! Head to Chapter 2 for the details on the ways you can age gracefully with a Mediterranean lifestyle.

Research shows that following a traditional Mediterranean diet significantly reduces the risk of heart disease and cancer, can help prevent or mitigate the problems associated with other chronic health conditions, and can offer all sorts of other benefits. The key word, however, is *traditional.* The Mediterranean region is changing, with faster-paced lifestyles and more modern conveniences. These changes bring with them an increased prevalence of heart disease and cancer. To get benefits from the Mediterranean diet, you need to follow the traditional diet.

Chapter 2

Opa! Reasons to Celebrate the Mediterranean Diet

In This Chapter
▶ Taking a close look at the powerful nutrients found in simple foods
▶ Highlighting the link between chronic conditions and the Mediterranean diet
▶ Looking and feeling your best with anti-aging tips

The Mediterranean diet has long been touted for providing health benefits, such as reducing coronary artery disease and decreasing the risk of some cancers. Including fresh vegetables and fruits, legumes, and healthy fats into your diet can help improve your health in many ways. And in addition to the health benefits, you're eating foods with full flavor. Thinking of bland or boring Greek or Italian food isn't easy.

This chapter highlights why this diet is full of health benefits by looking at some of the main nutrients found in Mediterranean eating and how characteristics of the diet itself, like portion sizes and the emphasis on savoring not only meals but life as well, make for a healthier, happier you.

A healthy diet, exercise, and stress management can significantly reduce your risk of certain diseases, but nothing can bring a guarantee. Genetic components also play a role with chronic diseases. However, if you have family history of heart disease, diabetes, or cancer, incorporating these lifestyle and diet changes into your daily life can help you decrease those risks.

Highlighting the Main Nutrients of the Mediterranean Diet

A plant-based diet such as the Mediterranean diet offers a plethora of nutrients that can help your body stay healthy. These plant foods are loaded with vitamins, minerals, antioxidants, phytochemicals, and healthy fats. The following sections highlight some of these key nutrients found in the foods associated with the Mediterranean coast.

These nutrients don't just benefit humans; the plant itself needs them so that it can grow and protect itself from the elements, bacteria, and other damage. Without nutrients, the plant can't grow or protect itself from oxidative damage or bacteria.

Fighting free radicals with antioxidants

Antioxidants are a key component of many plant foods that help slow down the process of oxidation (when your body's cells burn oxygen). This slowing decreases the amount of *free radicals,* or unstable molecules, that cause damage to your cells, tissues, and DNA. (Think about a sliced apple. Before you know it, the exposed flesh turns from white to brown. This browning occurs because of oxidation.)

Antioxidants are a crucial part of your diet because you can't avoid oxidation all together. Consider the many contaminants — car exhaust, sunlight, unhealthy foods, and air pollution, for example — that you're exposed to during a typical day. These types of exposures can cause free radicals to gain speed in your body, damaging everything in their path and leaving you at greater risk of chronic conditions like heart disease and cancer.

Eating a diet high in antioxidants such as vitamin C, vitamin E, and beta-carotene means better protection for your body and overall health. Go back to that sliced apple for a moment. If you brush the apple slice with orange juice or lemon juice right after you slice it, the flesh will stay whiter longer because of the antioxidant vitamin C in the juice.

The ATTICA study in the September 2005 issue of the *American Journal of Clinical Nutrition* measured the total antioxidant capacity of men and women in Greece. It found that the participants who followed a traditional Mediterranean diet had an 11 percent higher antioxidant capacity than those who didn't adhere to a traditional diet. The findings also showed that the participants who followed the traditional diet the most had 19 percent lower oxidized LDL (bad) cholesterol concentrations, showing a benefit in reducing heart disease.

You don't have to look far or even cook that much to get antioxidants into your diet. You can find plenty of antioxidants in fruits and vegetables. By eating five to eight servings of fruits and vegetables a day, you can take advantage of produces' antioxidants. Table 2-1 identifies some common foods, including lots of fruits and veggies, that are rich in certain antioxidants.

Table 2-1	Common Foods Containing Antioxidants		
Antioxidant	**Fruit**	**Vegetable**	**Nuts, Seeds, Spices**
Vitamin C	Cantaloupe, grapefruit, guava, lemons, oranges, pineapple, strawberries, tangerines	Asparagus, broccoli, cauliflower, green and red bell peppers, spinach, kale, collard greens, tomatoes	Chestnuts
Vitamin E	Apricots, avocadoes, cranberries, guava, nectarines, pomegranates	Mustard greens, Swiss chard, spinach, turnip and collard greens	Almonds, peanuts, sunflower seeds
Beta carotene	Apricots, cantaloupe, cherries, grapefruit, peaches, plums, tangerines	Broccoli, carrots, kale, spinach, turnip and collard greens; romaine lettuce	Cilantro, pistachios, pumpkin seeds

Should you supplement? Although you've likely heard the news that antioxidants found in foods promote good health, scientists are still researching whether taking supplements such as beta carotene, vitamin C, vitamin E, or other antioxidant blends can replace eating the real thing. Research has provided a great deal of information about many individual nutrients and their impacts on health, but researchers still don't have the answers to many questions, such as how much of a supplement is enough and whether supplemented antioxidants have the same effect working on their own as the natural ones do working with accompanying nutrients. Another supplement concern is that taking high doses of antioxidants may actually cause the antioxidants to work as *pro-oxidants* that promote rather than neutralize oxidation. The bottom line is that eating whole foods is still your best bet to combat diseases and live your healthiest life. As noted throughout the book, folks in the Mediterranean eat scads of produce, and this type of food intake is one of the reasons you see more longevity in people who live in this region.

Understanding phytochemicals

Besides vitamins and minerals, plants also contain *phytochemicals,* chemicals that offer your body healthful benefits. A plant-based diet high in fruits, vegetables, and legumes can provide you with an increased amount and variety of phytochemicals, helping to promote heart health and working to prevent certain cancers.

Research in this area is relatively new and is uncovering a whole side of previously unknown health benefits. To date, certain phytochemicals have been shown to work as antioxidants (see the previous section), contain anti-inflammatory properties, and promote heart health.

Phytochemicals provide the pigment to your fruits and vegetables, so you can literally know which class of phytochemicals you're consuming simply by noting the color you're eating. Table 2-2 shows a few specific health benefits found in each color.

Table 2-2	Potential Health Benefits of Foods by Color	
Color	*Health Benefits*	*Foods*
Blue/purple	A lower risk of some cancers; improved memory; and healthy aging	Blueberries, eggplant, purple grapes, and plums
Green	A lower risk of some cancers; healthy vision; and strong bones and teeth	Broccoli, green peppers, honeydew melon, kiwi, salad greens, and spinach
Red	A lower risk of heart disease and some cancers, and improved memory function	Pink watermelon, red bell peppers, and strawberries
White	A lower risk of heart disease and some cancers	Bananas, garlic, and onions
Yellow/orange	A lower risk of heart disease and some cancers; healthy vision; and a stronger immune system	Carrots, oranges, yellow and orange bell peppers, and yellow watermelon

Vitamin D: Getting a little of the sunshine vitamin

Your body gets vitamin D, otherwise known as the sunshine vitamin, both from food sources and from exposure to sunlight. The scientific community has been buzzing in the last ten years about the health benefits of vitamin D. Research shows this vitamin can help protect against osteoporosis, reduce the risk of coronary artery disease, decrease the risk of certain cancers, and lower the risk of infectious diseases such as the common flu.

People in the Mediterranean may be healthier because they have strong levels of the vitamin. One theory suggests that they're exposed to more sunlight — specifically, the ultraviolet B rays that are responsible for producing vitamin D — because of the region's location near the equator and because the people are outside more often walking, gardening, working, or enjoying family and friends.

To produce vitamin D, you want exposure to sunlight for 15 minutes each day with no sunscreen (sunscreen blocks up to 90 percent of vitamin D production). Of course, unprotected sun exposure increases the risk of skin cancer, so you have to weigh the good with the bad.

Many people, including those who have darker skin tones, are overweight, are older, or live in northern climates, don't make enough vitamin D from the sun. Fortunately, you can get vitamin D from a few foods, such as fish, fortified cereals, and fortified milk. Food sources are limited, so you mostly need to depend on sun exposure to get the proper amounts.

In 2010, the Institute of Medicine released a report recommending the following daily intake of vitamin D:

- ✔ **People ages 1 to 70:** 600 IU (international units) a day
- ✔ **People over the age of 70:** 800 IU (international units) a day

Many people need to add a supplement to ensure they're getting the daily dose they need, but don't try to guess how much you need; taking too much vitamin D can have harmful consequences. Discuss your needs with your physician.

Choosing healthy fats

The Mediterranean diet is lower in omega-6 polyunsaturated fats and saturated fats than most people's diets are; it's also higher in healthy fats, such as monounsaturated fats and omega-3 polyunsaturated fats. The higher percentage of monounsaturated fats found in the Mediterranean diet is associated with a lower risk of heart disease, lower cholesterol levels, decreased inflammation in the body, and better insulin function and blood sugar control.

You find monounsaturated fats in foods such as olive oil, avocadoes, and certain nuts. Polyunsaturated fatty acids are in corn, safflower, soybean, sesame, and sunflower oils and in seafood. Saturated fatty acids appear in animal-based foods such as meat, poultry, butter, and dairy products, as well as in coconut and palm oils.

Omega-3 fatty acids are one of the big contributors to the health benefits of the Mediterranean diet, and many people don't get enough of them. Research shows that omega-3s help reduce inflammation, which is specifically important for those with inflammatory diseases such as arthritis, cardiovascular disease, or inflammatory bowel disease. These fats are also shown to be helpful for immune system function, behavioral issues such as attention deficit (hyperactivity) disorder, mood disorders such as depression, and prevention of Alzheimer's disease.

Omega-6 fatty acids occur abundantly in the diet through sources such as grains, nuts, and legumes as well as sunflower, safflower, sesame, and corn oils, and animal protein. Omega-6 fats lower cholesterol, help keep the blood from clotting, and support skin health. Both omega-3 and omega-6 fats are considered essential, which means your body doesn't make them and needs to get them from your diet.

Your omega-6 intake should be higher than your omega-3 intake. Experts say the ratio to shoot for is about 4 parts omega-6 and 1 part omega-3. The big trouble begins when the balance between omega-3s and omega-6s gets out of whack. A diet too high in omega-6 fatty acids and too low in omega-3 fatty acids can promote conditions of chronic inflammation, including atherosclerosis, arthritis, and inflammatory bowel disease. Preliminary research also shows a possible connection to obesity, depression, dyslexia, and hyperactivity. This out-of-balance fat intake is very common in the American diet (with a ratio of 20 omega-6s to 1 omega-3) and less common in a Mediterranean-style diet.

Rebalance your diet by incorporating more sources of omega-3s, such as fresh herbs, canola oil, walnuts, flaxseeds, and cold-water fish (such as salmon, herring, and sturgeon), into your meals. You can also find products (such as eggs) fortified with omega 3s. Limit other sources of animal proteins (such as beef, poultry, unfortified eggs, and pork) by reducing your portion sizes to 2 to 3 ounces.

You can also repair the balance by replacing your cooking oils with olive oil, which is high in a third fat called omega-9 fatty acids. Your body can make omega-9s on its own, but adding more of them to your diet can help you lower your omega-6 intake.

Boosting your fiber intake

Fiber is what you may call the "roughage" found in plants. Your body doesn't digest fiber like it does nutrients; fiber goes through your gastrointestinal tract intact. This process has a bigger impact on health than you may think; its very important roles include the following:

✔ Helps maintain a healthy gastrointestinal tract

✔ Lowers total cholesterol and bad cholesterol levels

✔ Slows the absorption of sugars you consume from carbohydrate foods, which helps keep blood sugar stable

✔ Acts as a natural appetite suppressant, helping you to feel full and satisfied after a meal

You can get all the fiber you need by eating the Mediterranean way, focusing on fruits, vegetables, whole grains, and legumes.

Reviewing Health Benefits Associated with the Mediterranean Diet

Before researchers began their numerous studies on the people in the Mediterranean region and their diets, plenty of people had observed the overall good health enjoyed by the people in the region. As the later studies made clear, these observations were backed by cold, hard data (you can read about several of these studies in Chapter 18). The following sections outline the ways that the Mediterranean diet improves health.

As protection against heart disease

The Mediterranean diet is most noticed in the scientific community for its effect on heart health. The first research focused on the Mediterranean diet started with a scientist named Ancel Keys and the Seven Countries Study. This study found that southern Europe had far fewer coronary deaths than northern Europe and the United States did, even when factoring in age, smoking, blood pressure, and physical activity. These results made researchers look more closely at the differences in dietary habits.

Recent research continues to show a correlation between a traditional Mediterranean diet and lower incidence of heart disease. According to a 2008 study published in the *British Medical Journal,* research showed a 9 percent decrease in deaths from coronary artery disease. A 2011 review of several studies covering 535,000 people that was published in the *Journal of the American College of Cardiology* reported that a traditional Mediterranean diet is associated with lower blood pressure, blood sugar, and triglyceride levels.

Many more studies have shown the heart health protection of a diet high in fruits, vegetables, legumes, wine, and seafood, which supports the idea that the Mediterranean diet is a healthy lifestyle. Undoubtedly you can expect more and more research on this topic in the future.

As a weapon against cancer

Another area of research on the Mediterranean diet has focused on the diet's effects on preventing and managing cancer. Specific components of the diet have been shown to provide cancer-preventing and cancer-fighting benefits:

- **Plant foods:** A diet high in plant foods such as fruits, vegetables, legumes, and nuts may provide cancer protection. The high amounts of phytochemicals in these foods provide unique properties that can help inhibit or slow tumor growth or simply protect your cells. Refer to the earlier section "Understanding phytochemicals" for details on these powerhouses.

- **Meat:** Beginning in 1976, researchers from the Harvard School of Public Health followed 88,000 healthy women and found that the risk of colon cancer was 2.5 times higher in women who ate beef, pork, or lamb daily compared with those who ate those meats once a month or less. They also found that the risk of getting colon cancer was directly correlated to the amount of meat eaten.

- **Olive oil:** A study of 26,000 Greek people published in the *British Journal of Cancer* showed that using more olive oil cut cancer risk by 9 percent.

In addition to these ingredient-specific studies, the diet as a whole has some promising research. A 2008 study review published in the *British Medical Journal* showed that following a traditional Mediterranean diet reduced the risk of dying from cancer by 9 percent. That same year, the *American Journal of Clinical Nutrition* published a study that showed that among post-menopausal women, those who followed a traditional Mediterranean diet were 22 percent less likely to develop breast cancer. Although more research is needed in this area, you can enjoy a Mediterranean diet and know that you're helping increase your odds against cancer.

As protection against diabetes

The foods in the Mediterranean diet tend to be low-glycemic foods. The *glycemic index* is a measurement given to carbohydrate-containing foods that shows how quickly they turn into blood sugar. High-glycemic foods create a quick, high blood sugar spike, while low-glycemic foods offer a slow blood sugar rise. A diet that provides this slow rise in blood sugar is best for those with diabetes, whose bodies can't manage a large influx of sugar normally.

Most vegetables, fruits, whole grains, and legumes (hallmarks of the Mediterranean diet) provide a much slower blood sugar response compared to white bread, white pasta, or sugary snacks. A 2009 study from the Second University of Naples in Italy published in the *Annals of Internal Medicine* found that diabetics who followed a Mediterranean diet instead of a low-fat diet had better glycemic control and were less likely to need diabetes medication.

The portion sizes in the Mediterranean diet can also make a significant difference for someone with diabetes. Starchy foods such as the whole grains found in cereals and breads can also make blood sugar rise if a person consumes too much of them, but the portion sizes associated with a Mediterranean pattern of eating are much lower and help keep total carbohydrate intake during the meal in check.

But the benefits don't stop at those who already have diabetes; this diet pattern may help you reduce your risk of getting the disease. The SUN cohort study from the University of Navarra, Spain, which involved more than 13,000 participants with no history of diabetes, showed that those participants who followed a Mediterranean-style diet were less likely to develop type 2 diabetes. What's more interesting about this study is that participants who had high risk factors for type 2 diabetes (including older age, family history of diabetes, and a history of smoking) and followed the diet pattern strictly had an 83 percent relative reduction for developing the disease.

As an anti-aging regimen

A Mediterranean lifestyle can also help you feel and look your best. Here are some of the ways you can age gracefully with a Mediterranean lifestyle:

- ✔ **Increased longevity:** The NIH-AARP Diet and Health Study published in the *Archives of Internal Medicine* in 2007 found that people who closely adhered to a Mediterranean-style diet were 12 to 20 percent less likely to die from cancer and all causes.

- ✔ **Wrinkle reduction:** A study published in the *Journal of the American College of Nutrition* in 2001 found that people who consumed a diet high in fruits, vegetables, nuts, legumes, and fish had less skin wrinkling. Of course, this area needs far more research, but eating healthy foods sure beats plastic surgery, right?

- ✔ **Smoother skin:** Eating a diet high in vitamin C foods, such as oranges, strawberries, and broccoli, plays an important role in the production of collagen, the skin's support structure. Refer to Table 2-1 earlier in the chapter for more vitamin C–rich foods.

✔ **Inflammation reduction:** Inflammation can affect your heart health, joints, and skin. Eating a diet high in anti-inflammatory foods such as cold-water fish, walnuts, flaxseeds, and fresh herbs can help keep you feeling your best.

✔ **Lowered Alzheimer's risk:** A 2006 study at Columbia University Medical Center showed that participants who followed a Mediterranean-style diet had 40 percent lower risk of Alzheimer's disease than those who didn't.

Because the Mediterranean diet focuses on a healthy lifestyle as well as consuming healthy foods and food portions, it offers other anti-aging benefits:

✔ **Bone density maintenance:** Moderate weight-bearing exercise such as walking or lifting weights can maintain good bone density, keeping your bones strong and helping you avoid bone fractures later in life.

✔ **Tension taming:** A good laugh reduces tension and stress in the body, leaving your muscles relaxed for up to 45 minutes. Stress can lead to depression, anxiety, high blood pressure, and heart disease, all of which contribute to aging and a reduced quality of life.

As a way of maintaining a healthy weight

Obesity, already at epidemic levels in the U.S., is becoming a major health problem around the world as globalization introduces more American-style eating patterns to other cultures: prepackaged convenience foods, large portion sizes, and food selections that are high in calories and fat. Although any diet in which you consume fewer calories than your body needs can result in weight loss, the particular foods that make up the Mediterranean diet, the way the foods are portioned and balanced, and the added focus on *how* you eat make maintaining a healthy weight — or losing weight — that much easier. The following sections explain why.

Considering calories without counting them

Calories are the amount of energy in the foods you eat and the amount of energy your body uses for daily activities. Your body constantly needs energy or fuel not only for daily activities such as cooking, cleaning, and exercising but also for basic biological functions. Everyone has a different metabolic rate that determines how quickly he or she burns calories and depends on factors such as age, genetics, gender, and physical fitness level.

At the end of the day, you can't lose weight if you eat more calories than you burn through daily activity and exercise. To lose weight, you have to create a calorie deficit, but you can do so without actually knowing how many calories you burn. All you have to do is make small changes to your lifestyle, such as reducing portion sizes to reduce your calorie intake and exercising more to increase how many calories you use.

Coffee's health benefits: Full of beans?

Coffee is a complex nutrition topic because it's a natural, plant-based food containing healthy antioxidants, which may be to thank for the lower rates of type 2 diabetes, Parkinson's disease, and dementia in coffee drinkers. However, the caffeine in coffee may increase blood pressure (though you can drink decaf to avoid this problem), and coffee in general may increase homocysteine levels, which is a risk factor for heart disease, regardless of the caffeine content. More research is needed to provide any definitive recommendations for or against caffeine and coffee, but enjoying it in moderation is likely the key.

Enjoying *espresso,* a form of concentrated coffee, is a tradition on the Mediterranean coast, but folks there tend to look at espresso as a morning drink only and often drink just one to two ounces of espresso a day (a stark contrast to many coffee-shop regulars in the United States). One ounce of espresso contains around 75 milligrams of caffeine, compared to 135 milligrams in one cup of coffee.

If you don't drink coffee, there is certainly no reason for you to start. If you're a coffee lover, enjoy your coffee, but try to limit yourself to one to two 8-ounce cups of coffee or one to two 1-ounce shots of espresso each day.

Without having some idea of your calorie intake level, however, you'll be in the dark about how much you're eating. That's where the Mediterranean diet comes into play. Instead of counting calories, you think about the kinds of foods you eat and the portion sizes of those foods. By adding more low-calorie fruits and vegetables to your diet and decreasing the portion size of higher-calorie foods like meats and grains, you can decrease your calorie level naturally. When you master this new way of eating, you can ensure you're eating the appropriate number of calories without having to account for every single one.

You can eat an appropriate number of calories just by properly balancing your plate's food make-up, controlling portions, and expending energy through fun activities. As an added bonus, these lower-calorie foods also help you feel more satisfied with your meal instead of feeling deprived. Here's how:

- **Simply changing the balance of the foods you eat makes a huge difference in your calorie intake:** In the United States, a traditional plate of food has a large piece of meat, a large serving of grains or potatoes, and a tiny amount of vegetable. By simply switching up your plate to include small portions of meat and grain, two to three vegetables, and perhaps a serving of legumes, you can easily save calories (in some cases, hundreds of them). For example, one 6-ounce chicken breast is around 276 calories. Decrease the serving size to 3 ounces, and the count drops to 138 calories. That one change saves 138 calories. A serving of vegetables (one-half cup cooked or 1 cup raw) is only 25 calories. By the time you put two to three of those servings on your plate, you've spent about 75 calories and don't have space for much else.

✔ **Paying attention to portion sizes is a far better way to decrease your calorie intake than counting calories.** Portion sizes in the Mediterranean are different than they are in the United States, which is one reason folks in the Mediterranean region tend to manage their weights more effectively. Although the U.S. serving-size guidelines are appropriate, few Americans actually follow them. Table 2-3 is a serving guide that can help you create smaller, appropriate portions and thus a lower-calorie plate; after you get the hang of it, eating the right portion size will be second nature, and you'll just know how much to put on your plate by eyeballing it.

Table 2-3	Serving Size Guide
Food	*Serving Size*
Grains	1 slice bread
	½ an English muffin, hamburger bun, or bagel
	⅓ cup rice
	½ cup cooked cereal, pasta, or other cooked grain
	¾ cup cold cereal
	One 6-inch tortilla
Other starchy carbohydrates	½ cup beans or lentils (these also contain protein)
Fruit	1 medium piece of fruit
	½ cup canned or sliced fruit
	6 ounces (¾ cup) 100 percent fruit juice
Vegetables	1 cup raw
	½ cup cooked
	6 ounces (¾ cup) 100 percent vegetable juice
Dairy	8 ounces of milk or yogurt
	⅓ cup cottage cheese
	1 ounce cheese
Protein	½ cup beans (beans are also high in carbs)
	2–4 ounces beef, poultry, pork, or fish (size of a deck of cards)
	1 ounce cheese
	1 egg
	1 ounce nuts
	1 tablespoon nut spreads (such as peanut butter, almond butter, and so on)

Food	Serving Size
Fats	⅛ of an avocado (2 tablespoons)
	1 teaspoon oil, butter, margarine, or mayonnaise
	2 teaspoon whipped butter
	8 olives
	1 tablespoon regular salad dressing
	2 tablespoons low-fat salad dressing

Increasing activity you love

Exercise is an important component to weight loss and health, especially with the Mediterranean diet. Exercise allows you to not only burn calories but also strengthen your heart, manage stress, and increase your energy level.

Starting an exercise program may be challenging for you — maybe the thought of going to a busy gym and running on a treadmill sounds more painful than a double root canal. Never fear; look to the Mediterranean. On the Mediterranean coast, the main focus on exercise is walking, working, and engaging in enjoyable activities instead of formalized exercise programs. That is, people walk to run errands; lift and carry groceries home; work in the yard; and enjoy fun activities like bike riding or swimming.

If starting an exercise program sounds difficult for you, find activities that you actually enjoy doing and look for ways to get out every day for a walk. The American College of Sports Medicine and the American Heart Association recommend getting 30 minutes of moderate exercise (you get your heart rate up but can still have a conversation) a day, five days a week for those who are 18 to 65 years old, as well as adding two days a week of strength-training exercises like lifting weights.

Suppressing your appetite effortlessly

Eating a Mediterranean-style diet is not only great for your health but can also work as a natural appetite suppressant to help manage your weight. When you eat the right balance of plant-based foods and healthy fats, your body works in a natural way to feel satisfied. Because you're full, you're not tempted (at least, not by your stomach) to snack on high-calorie junk food a short while after your last meal. Following are the three main reasons a Mediterranean diet helps to control your appetite:

✔ **Loading up on fiber:** Fiber, found in fruits, vegetables, whole grains, and legumes, provides bulk and slows down digestion to help you feel full for a longer period of time. With the Mediterranean diet, you consume much more fiber-rich food with each meal and snack, which can make you feel satisfied all day. These high-fiber foods also make you chew a little longer, helping you to slow down at mealtime.

Your brain takes 20 minutes to register that you're full, which is longer than many people spend eating a meal. As a result, your brain may give you the okay to keep eating because it doesn't realize yet that you've actually eaten enough to be full. Chewing more helps you to slow down and reach that 20-minute mark.

✔ **Turning on your fullness hormones:** Appetite is controlled by an intricate dance of hormones that trigger the feelings of hunger and fullness. As noted in the earlier section "As protection against diabetes," the Mediterranean diet is naturally high in low-glycemic foods, those carbohydrate-containing foods that illicit a lower blood sugar spike. Low-glycemic foods may just help kick in your fullness response.

Feeling biologically full and psychologically satisfied with your meal are two very different things that are often hard to distinguish. Biological fullness occurs in your stomach, where you feel hungry, neutral, or comfortably full. Feeling psychologically satisfied is in your brain; you want to eat more because it tastes so good! Overindulging once in awhile because something is so tasty is completely normal, but when you consistently ignore your fullness cues and eat until you're psychologically satisfied, you consume too many calories far too often. If you fall into this trap, tell yourself you can have more of the food later in the day or even tomorrow. Heck, you can even make this meal again and again so that you can enjoy it every week.

One of the first signs of dehydration is hunger, so when you feel hungry, even though you just ate a short time ago, grab a glass of water, wait 15 minutes, and see how you feel.

Controlling food cravings

Keeping your blood sugar stable throughout the day is a good strategy to help manage food cravings. To do so, follow these suggestions:

✔ **Make sure you don't skip meals or wait longer than five hours to eat.** Eat a meal or snack every three to five hours.

✔ **Eat protein-rich foods and a bit of fat.** Foods such as fish, beans, nuts, or eggs eaten with a bit of fat help slow down your digestion.

✔ **Eat high-fiber fruits, vegetables, grains, and legumes with each meal and snack.** You don't have to eat these foods all at once, but include some combination of them throughout the day.

✔ **Manage your stress hormones.** Stress releases hormones that trigger the "fight or flight" response (where your body gears up its energy levels for a big event like fighting or fleeing) and kick on your hunger hormones. First, manage stress levels, a priority in traditional Mediterranean life: exercise, get enough sleep, drink water, practice deep breathing, meditate, and relax. Second, when you feel a craving, choose a low-glycemic snack and include some omega-3 fatty acids. A good snack is some tuna fish spread on whole-grain crackers. This combination can help you get the fuel your body is craving but also help your central nervous system calm down.

Mastering the art of mindful eating

A traditional Mediterranean style of eating engages regularly in mindful eating, something that many have completely lost track of. With *mindful eating,* you can manage your weight by paying attention to your internal body cues. Yes, your own body has a very sophisticated weight management system built in that includes hormones that tell you when you should eat and when to stop (see the earlier section "Suppressing your appetite effortlessly" for details). The problem is that too many people often ignore that reflex. These suggestions can help you refocus on these internal cues and become completely satisfied with what you're eating:

✔ **Slow down:** A good goal is to spend at least 20 to 30 minutes eating your larger meals. As noted earlier in the chapter, this time frame gives your biological system time to let you know when you're full. Plus, it allows you to sit and enjoy your food. Use these tips to help you slow down at meal time:

- Set your fork down between bites to begin retraining yourself how to slow down while you eat. Alternatively, take a deep breath and count to ten before each bite. Don't worry — you don't have to do this forever, just until you've learned how to pace yourself.

- Have great table discussions with your family and friends. Ask a question about everyone's day or talk about current events.

- Take some time to be grateful for what you have.

- Make meal time a television-, computer-, and phone-free zone to avoid mindless eating.

✔ **Enjoy food to its fullest:** When you eat, take time to enjoy every aspect of your food. Before you dig into any food, smell the flavors coming from it. Taste each and every flavor: during each bite, let the food sit in your mouth. Chew it slowly and take pleasure in the freshness and the many tastes that roll across your taste buds.

Part II
Common Ailments and the Positive Effects of the Mediterranean Diet

Health Goal	Follow This Mediterranean Diet Principle
Reduce the risk and progression of heart disease	Swap out butter and limit red meat and full-fat dairy products in favor of olive oil, nuts, seeds, avocado, and fish
	Eat whole grains, fruits and veggies, nuts, seeds, and legumes to lower cholesterol and maintain a healthy weight
	Drink red wine in moderation, which protects the blood vessel lining in your heart
	Maintain a healthy weight
Maintain a healthy blood pressure and lower your risk of stroke	Make olive oil your primary fat source
	Consume minimally processed foods like fresh fruits, vegetables, nuts, seeds, and whole grains
	Remain or become active
Lower your risk of diabetes or mitigate its severity	Eat more whole grains and fiber-full carbohydrates, like quinoa, bulgur, and barley
	Use extra virgin olive oil as your main source of fat
	Eat foods rich in omega-3 and monounsaturated fatty acids, flavonoids, and carotenoids
	Maintain a healthy weight
Maintain a healthy weight or lose weight	Focus on real rather than processed and packaged foods, specifically plant-based foods, lean proteins, and healthy fats
	Reduce or eliminate fast foods, foods that are high in sugar, and high-fat meats and dairy
	Adopt an active lifestyle
Reduce your risk of colorectal, breast, and other cancers	Eat less meat and get your protein from fish, eggs, nuts, seeds, and whole grains
	Eat more fruits and veggies
	Make olive oil your fat of choice

Not smoking is one of the best things you can do for your health. Find out how to quit at www.dummies.com/extras/mediterraneandiet.

In this part . . .

✔ Discover the key symptoms and causes of heart disease and see how incorporating healthy fats, plant-based foods, and red wine into your diet can help you avoid the conditions that lead to heart disease and heart attacks.

✔ Learn how both the dietary and lifestyle components of the Mediterranean diet help keep your blood pressure within normal limits and lower your risk for stroke.

✔ Find out how whole grains, olive oil, and the predominance of fruits and vegetables result in improved blood sugar control and reduced insulin resistance, can eliminate the need for diabetes medication, and have been shown to prevent diabetes even in at-risk populations.

✔ Note how the diet's focus on whole, unprocessed foods, healthy fats, and an active lifestyle helps you lose excess weight and maintain a healthy weight.

✔ Figure out how nutrients in the Mediterranean diet help prevent cancer, improve lifespans, and help cancer patients overcome the affects of chemotherapy and radiation.

Chapter 3

Heart Disease and Heart Attackackackack: What You Ought to Know by Now

• •

In This Chapter

▶ Taking a quick look at how the heart works

▶ Familiarizing yourself with heart problems and risk factors

▶ Taking steps to protect your heart

▶ Connecting benefits of the Mediterranean diet to your heart's health

• •

T he heart is so magical for us. We tell loved ones that they live inside our hearts. We say that someone with enormous courage has "tremendous heart." Lovers are said to die of a broken heart. We all have an emotional attachment to this miraculous pump that we simply do not feel for any other organ. Would you ever think about your lungs or kidneys or pancreas in this way? Of course not. Humans seem to have a built-in sense of the heart's importance. And cardiovascular disease in all its forms is the biggest threat to our hearts.

The heart captivates our imagination for good reason — human health, daily performance, and life itself depend on the heart — which is why it's so important to take care of it. This chapter provides general information on how the heart works, describes the kinds of problems that can occur, identifies risk factors for heart disease, and tells you how the Mediterranean diet, while certainly not a cure-all, can be one positive step you can take to keep your remarkable heart healthy.

Taking a Closer Look at the Heart

Despite the emotional energy we attach to our hearts and the heart's crucial importance to life itself, most people are pretty ignorant about the heart and how it works. You know that your life depends on your heart. What you may not know is that the average adult heart is about the size of a clenched fist and weighs less than a pound. The heart is the engine that keeps your body functioning. When disease or injury strikes the heart, the body's ability to function declines as the heart's ability declines. Read on for more information on how the heart works.

Note: The following sections offer a very simplified explanation of the heart's structure and function. For detailed explanations of this vital organ, the diseases that can afflict it, and the treatment options available, both through lifestyle modifications and medical interventions, check out *Heart Disease For Dummies,* by Dr. James Rippe (Wiley).

The heart as a pump

The heart, shown in Figure 3-1, is a magnificent four-chambered pump that has two jobs:

- Pumping blood to the lungs to get oxygen
- Pumping the oxygenated blood to the rest of the body

To fulfill these tasks, the heart has a left and a right side, each with one main pumping chamber called a *ventricle* located in the lower part of it. Sitting above the left and right ventricles are two small booster pumps called *atria* (or *atrium*, when you're talking about just one). The right ventricle pumps deoxygenated blood, which returns from the body through veins and the right atrium, out into the lungs where it receives a new supply of oxygen. The blood then returns to the heart, first entering the left atrium and then the left ventricle. The left ventricle pumps oxygenated blood through the arterial system out to the rest of the body where it feeds every vital organ — in fact, every single living cell — you have.

In the average adult, the heart pumps 5 quarts of blood per minute at rest and 25 to 30 quarts per minute at maximum effort. In highly trained athletes working at maximum effort, the amount of blood pumped per minute can run as high as 40 quarts.

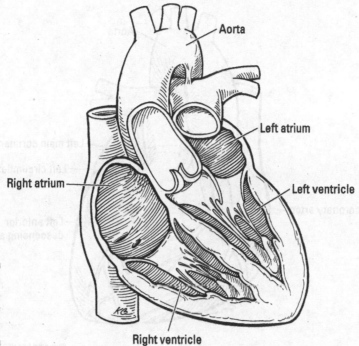

Aorta

Left atrium

Right atrium

Left ventricle

Figure 3-1:
The four
chambers of
the heart.

Right ventricle

Illustration by Kathryn Born, MA

The coronary arteries

Three large coronary arteries and their many branches supply blood to the heart. As you can see in Figure 3-2, two coronary arteries branch off one main trunk, which is called the *left main coronary artery*. One of these branches runs down the front of the heart, so in medspeak, it is naturally called the *left anterior descending artery*. (*Anterior* is just a fancy word for front.) The second branch of the left main coronary artery circles around and supplies the side wall of the heart, so it is called the *left circumflex artery*. The third main coronary artery, which typically comes off of a separate trunk vessel, is called the *right coronary artery*. It supplies the back and bottom walls of the heart.

Significant narrowing of any of these coronary arteries causes angina, a symptom typically characterized as chest pain. (You can read more about angina in the later section "Angina.") A small or minor blockage of an artery can spontaneously rupture or tear. This results in a blood clot forming that blocks blood flow completely, causing a heart attack.

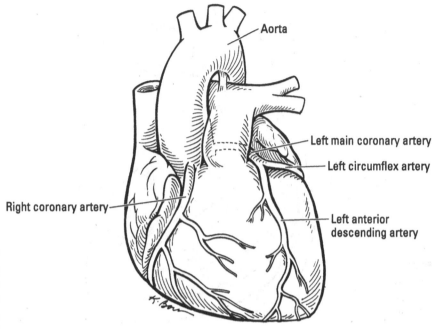

Aorta

Left main coronary artery

Left circumflex artery

Right coronary artery

Left anterior descending artery

Figure 3-2:
The coronary arteries.

Illustration by Kathryn Born, MA

Sliding down the slippery slope toward heart disease

When all parts of the heart and cardiovascular system are healthy and functioning well together, it is a beautiful system. But the heart is a muscle. And like any muscle, it works best when you keep it in shape and avoid injury.

The conditioned heart

A conditioned heart is stronger and better able to meet the demands the body places on it. Human bodies were designed to be in motion. And the motion of physical activity keeps the heart well tuned, the benefits of which are numerous:

✔ Literally hundreds of studies have shown that individuals who adopt the simple habit of daily physical activity substantially reduce their risk of developing various heart problems, most notably coronary artery disease (CAD).

✔ The conditioned heart enables individuals to accomplish the activities of daily living with comfort and without running out of breath and energy.

✔ The more conditioned the heart, the lower the resting heart rate, and the less work the heart has to do in a lifetime.

✔ Studies show that, with appropriate activity, hearts damaged by disease or injury can regain conditioning that enhances health and function and may even contribute to the reversal of some aspects of disease.

The deconditioned heart

In contrast to the active individual, the individual who leads a sedentary lifestyle can actually experience a deconditioned heart. The deconditioned heart is less efficient at doing its work and has to work harder to get adequate blood flow throughout the body. You're a prime candidate for a deconditioned heart if you answer "yes" to these questions or others like them:

✔ Do you avoid the stairs because climbing two or three flights leaves you extremely short of breath?

✔ Do you circle a parking lot numerous times looking for a space right in front of the store to make sure that you don't have to walk much?

✔ Do you watch sports on television rather than participate in them with friends and family?

✔ On a nice day, do you pop a DVD into the player rather than take a walk?

For many people, a deconditioned heart is the first step in a slow slide down the long slope toward a sick heart.

The diseased heart

A sedentary lifestyle coupled with unhealthy practices such as poor nutrition, weight gain, cigarette smoking, or certain other health conditions, such as high blood pressure, high cholesterol, or diabetes, can severely alter the basic cardiac structures. A short list of the things that can go wrong includes blocked arteries, high blood pressure, angina, heart attack, heart failure, and sudden death. The bottom line: Many of the cardiac problems that people experience are brought on by years of neglect and failure to abide by even the most basic of cardiac-healthy lifestyle principles. (Nature makes a few mistakes, too, but even in those cases, personal choices often complicate the problem.)

The good news is that even if you've been diagnosed as at-risk for heart disease or as having it, and even if you've experienced specific heart problems, paying attention to the basic principles of a cardiac-healthy lifestyle in conjunction with the medications and procedures of your treatment plan can help you turn things around.

The Rogues Gallery: From Heart Conditions to Heart Failure

Heart disease is public health enemy number one in America. In one or another of its manifestations, heart disease touches virtually every family in the United States. Consider these startling facts:

- Almost 60 million Americans — almost one in every four — have one or more types of heart disease.

- Heart disease and stroke cause more than one of every two deaths — more deaths than all other diseases combined.

- An individual is more than 10 times more likely to die of heart disease than in an accident and more than 30 times as likely to die of heart disease than of AIDS.

- Heart disease is an equal-opportunity killer. It is the leading cause of death in men and women and all ethnic and racial groups in the United States.

- If money is the most important thing in your life, you might like to know that the yearly estimated cost of cardiovascular disease in the United States is $286.5 billion.

As startling as these statistics may be, you can take charge of your heart health. The following sections briefly explain the different kinds of problems that can afflict your heart.

Coronary artery disease

Coronary artery disease (CAD) is the slow, progressive narrowing of the three main arteries (and their branches) that supply blood to the heart. This narrowing of the arteries gradually starves the heart muscle of the oxygenated blood that it needs to function properly. A lack of adequate blood supply to the heart typically produces symptoms that range from angina to heart attack or sudden death.

Narrowing arteries that are characteristic of CAD result from the gradual buildup of fatty deposits called *plaque* on their interior walls. These deposits are made up of cholesterol, other fats, cellular wastes, platelets, calcium, and other substances. These deposits typically start with fatty streaks and grow to large bumps that distort the artery and block its interior where the blood must flow. Some plaques are stable, and others are unstable or vulnerable to cracking or rupturing, which often leads to an artery-blocking blood clot and subsequent heart attack.

Atherosclerosis, the most common medical term for CAD, comes from two Greek words — athero (paste, gruel) and sclerosis (hardness) — that may give you a graphic image of hardened sludge. Not a pretty picture, is it?

Biological factors that contribute to the development of CAD are present from birth and perform vital functions that enable the human body to grow and resist infection. As a consequence, all human beings are born with the potential to develop CAD. In fact, the first visible signs of CAD, fatty streaks on inner artery walls, frequently occur in children, teens, and young adults. Decades and the presence of various risk factors are required for the streaks to develop into intermediate (moderate-sized, symptomless) and advanced (larger, symptom-producing) plaques. Figure 3-3 illustrates the typical but gradual development and progression of CAD.

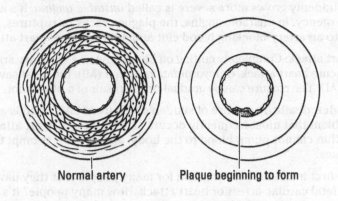

Normal artery   Plaque beginning to form

Figure 3-3:
The process
of coronary
artery
disease.

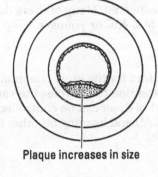

Plaque increases in size   Large plaque has formed

Illustration by Kathryn Born, MA

Recognizing the symptoms and manifestations of CAD

Because every person is an individual, physical responses to progressive coronary artery disease vary. Not every individual with CAD has every manifestation and symptom of the condition. Individuals likewise experience specific symptoms in different ways. But these manifestations are typical:

- ✔ **Nothing:** Many people can have significant CAD but experience no discomfort or other sign of the disease. That's why this condition is known in medicine as *silent ischemia*. *Ischemia* means lack of blood flow. People with diabetes are particularly susceptible to silent ischemia, but others can have it, too.

- ✔ **Angina:** More formally known as *angina pectoris*, angina is typified by temporary chest pain, usually during exertion. This pain usually is felt as a tightness or uncomfortable feeling across the chest or up to the neck and jaw, not as a sharp stab. Angina also may have other manifestations.

- ✔ **Unstable angina:** Chest pain that is new, occurs when you're at rest, or suddenly grows more severe is called *unstable angina*. It's a medical emergency. In unstable angina, the plague cracks or ruptures, often leading to an artery-blocking blood clot and, ultimately, a heart attack.

- ✔ **Heart attack:** Completely cutting off blood flow to a coronary artery causes an acute heart attack, or *myocardial infarction* (MI), the most severe result of CAD. The closure can be gradual or the result of a blood clot.

- ✔ **Sudden death:** The cause of sudden death from CAD often is a rhythm problem that most frequently occurs as a result of a heart attack. The rhythm cannot pump blood to the body, and without prompt CPR, death ensues.

The first indication or symptom for many people that they have CAD is a fatal cardiac arrest or heart attack. How many people? It's hard to say exactly, but 250,000 sudden cardiac deaths occur each year, and the American Heart Association indicates that about half of all deaths caused by CAD are sudden and unexpected. Many of these deaths happen to younger people in their 50s, 40s, or younger.

Identifying who's at risk for CAD

In this section, you discover the risk factors for the most common form of CAD, or atherosclerosis. Paying close attention to the roles the various risk factors play and remembering that most of them can be controlled go a long way toward slowing or even reversing CAD and heading off other heart problems down the road.

Those with hypertension

Elevated blood pressure, or *hypertension*, represents a substantial risk for developing CAD and stroke. Hypertension appears to be particularly dangerous in terms of the likelihood of developing a stroke. (For an in-depth discussion of hypertension and stroke, see Chapter 4.)

Hypertension is extremely common in the United States, probably because of the nutritional habits, propensity to gain weight, and sedentary lifestyle of most Americans. The good news is that daily habits and practices, such as appropriate weight control, sound nutrition, and regular physical activity, can profoundly diminish the likelihood of your ever developing hypertension in the first place and can significantly contribute to the effective treatment of elevated blood pressure.

Those with high cholesterol

By now, almost everyone knows having a high cholesterol level in your blood is a bad thing. When it comes to being at risk of developing CAD, however, an elevated level of blood cholesterol is one of a number of lipid problems (problems with fats in the blood) that significantly elevate your risk of heart disease. The abnormalities that are particularly dangerous include elevated total cholesterol, elevated "bad" (LDL) cholesterol, low "good" (HDL) cholesterol, elevated triglycerides, or any combination of the four.

The good news is that by following appropriate lifestyle measures and, in some instances, using effective medicines that now are available, this risk factor for CAD can be effectively managed.

Tobacco users

Cigarette smoking (and the use of other tobacco products) is the leading cause of premature death in the United States each year, claiming more than 400,000 lives.

The health consequences of cigarette smoking are severe. Smoking

- ✓ Triples the risk of developing heart disease and increases the risk of developing lung cancer by a whopping 3,000 percent
- ✓ Tends to lower "good" (HDL) cholesterol

In an otherwise bleak picture, the outstanding good news is that stopping smoking lowers the risk of developing CAD and significantly improves the health outlook for individuals who have heart disease; can add two to three years to your life expectancy; and improves blood lipids. In one study, LDL cholesterol decreased more than 5 percent and HDL cholesterol increased more than 3 percent in individuals who stopped cigarette smoking.

Quitting is so important (and so tough) that you want to increase your chances of success by stocking your arsenal with strategies that give you the ways and means — and support — to stamp out smoking in your life. Go online to www.dummies.com/extras/mediterraneandiet to find one such strategy.

Those who are physically inactive

In 1994, faced with overwhelming evidence, the American Heart Association added the first new major factor in 25 years — a physically inactive lifestyle — to the list of risks for developing CAD. Physical inactivity is defined as a major factor, in part, because it also contributes significantly to a number of the other major risk factors, such as high blood pressure, perhaps elevated blood cholesterol, and often obesity. But if you get off your duff and get active, you can turn this sad picture around. A physically active lifestyle not only reduces the specific risk that inactivity poses for heart disease, but it also helps lessen or eradicate several of the other major risk factors for heart disease.

For an easy way to get active, head online to www.dummies.com/extras/ mediterraneandiet, where you'll find a strategy to get yourself walking 10,000 steps a day.

Those who are obese or overweight

In 1998, obesity joined the list of major independent risk factors for developing CAD. Like physical inactivity, obesity also contributes to many other risk factors, including hypertension and elevated cholesterol, and other abnormal lipid levels.

Being obese increases the risk of CAD in a number of different ways. First, obesity interacts negatively with many other risk factors for developing CAD, such as high blood pressure, type 2 diabetes, and cholesterol problems. Second, obese people are particularly susceptible to a clustering of risk factors. In fact, obese individuals are 70 percent more likely to be affected by at least one other risk factor for heart disease and 50 percent more likely to be affected by at least two other risk factors for heart disease. Third, obesity serves as a forerunner to dangerous lipid abnormalities, such as elevated blood triglycerides and LDL cholesterol levels, that increase the risk of heart disease. Carrying extra weight around the abdomen (sometimes called *abdominal obesity* or *apple-shaped obesity*) is particularly dangerous in terms of its risk of coronary heart disease.

If you're overweight, regardless of whether you have heart disease, you need to make a point of talking to your doctor about whether you show signs of having other risk factors for heart disease in addition to obesity. The odds are that you do. And if you've been diagnosed with heart disease and are overweight, then be sure to discuss these issues with your physician. Weight loss in and of itself is a highly effective way of reducing multiple risk factors for heart disease. Chapter 6 has the details.

Those with diabetes mellitus

Diabetes represents a significant risk factor for coronary heart disease. Individuals with diabetes often have multiple blood lipid abnormalities, including elevated blood triglycerides, elevated LDL cholesterol, and depressed HDL cholesterol. Having this particular constellation of lipid abnormalities spells triple trouble!

Risk factors you can't modify

All the risk factors mentioned previously in this chapter are ones that you can change, even if doing so is hard. If you smoke, for example, you can stop. If you're overweight or sedentary, you can shed the extra pounds and make physical activity part of your daily regimen. There are three risk factors, however, that you can't modify: your age, gender, and family history:

✔ **Age:** Age is considered a significant risk factor for CAD for men who are older than 45 and for women who are older than 55 or have undergone premature menopause.

✔ **Gender:** Men are more likely to develop CAD than women. Furthermore, the onset of symptoms of CAD typically occurs ten years later in women than in men; however, CAD remains the number-one killer in *both* men and women in the United States. CAD

becomes particularly prevalent in women after menopause. After age 65, men and women have approximately the same risk for developing CAD.

✔ **Family history:** CAD tends to occur more frequently in some families than in others. Coming from a family in which a diagnosed heart attack or a sudden death before age 55 in males or age 65 in females occurred increases your risk. Having a first-degree relative (father, mother, brother, or sister) who fits this description also qualifies as a risk factor.

Having one or more of these non-modifiable risk factors makes it particularly important that you pay close attention to the risk factors that you *can* modify.

For reasons that to date are not totally clear, women with diabetes have an even greater risk of developing heart disease than men with diabetes. Recent compelling research also indicates that individuals who have some degree of insulin resistance or glucose intolerance — test results that put them in the "prediabetic" category — also have elevated risk of heart disease.

In addition to working with your physician, you can help control your diabetes by losing weight if you're overweight, engaging in regular physical activity, and adopting proper nutritional habits. Chapter 5 has more on diabetes.

Angina

When coronary artery disease progresses enough to significantly diminish the blood flow to heart tissue, it produces angina pectoris, which is commonly called simply *angina*. Angina typically is a discomfort felt in the chest, often beneath the breastbone (or sternum) or in nearby areas such as the neck, jaw, back, or arms.

- ✔ Individuals often describe the chest discomfort as a "squeezing sensation," "vicelike," "constricting," or " a heavy pressure on the chest." It is commonly referred to simply as a "chest pain."

- ✔ Angina often is brought on by physical exertion or strong emotions and typically is relieved within several minutes by resting or using nitroglycerin.

- ✔ Some individuals may experience angina as a symptom different from chest discomfort or in addition to it. Shortness of breath, faintness, or fatigue may also be manifestations of angina, although if chest pain is absent, they may be called *anginal equivalents*.

- ✔ When chest pain occurs at rest, it usually is classified as *unstable angina*. With unstable angina, the plaques often appear structurally weak and may be easily ruptured or torn by a number of forces, ranging from the normal flow of blood at high stress points in the arterial system to sudden pressures such as suddenly increased blood pressure from exertion.

Angina usually does not damage the heart. It is a temporary condition — the usual episode lasts only five to ten minutes. The discomfort that comes with angina is your heart's way of getting your attention. It occurs when you ask your heart to work harder, and it therefore demands more blood — for instance, when you're walking briskly or running, climbing a hill or stairs, having sex, or doing housework or yard work. Strong emotions such as fear or anger also can trigger an episode. The discomfort makes you stop and rest, slowing the heart and lessening its demand for blood. Alternatively, most people with angina take a nitroglycerin tablet under the tongue when they have an angina attack. The nitroglycerin dilates the coronary arteries, enabling blood flow to the heart to increase.

Any discomfort that lasts longer that five to ten minutes or doesn't stop with rest may be a heart attack and needs to be treated as an emergency.

Heart attacks

A heart attack occurs when one of the three coronary arteries that supply oxygen-rich blood to the heart muscle becomes severely or totally blocked, usually by a blood clot. When the heart muscle doesn't receive enough oxygenated blood, it begins to die. The severity of the heart attack depends on how much of the heart is injured or dies when the attack occurs.

Understanding the causes of a heart attack

Heart attack almost always is caused when a blood clot forms at the site of an existing fatty plaque that has ruptured or broken open. Thus, individuals are at much higher risk for heart attack if they

- ✔ Have a history of CAD

- ✔ Have experienced previous bouts of angina

- ✔ Have suffered a previous heart attack

The blockage that triggers a heart attack usually is caused by an acute blood clot. Most acute blood clots occur when one of the plaques or fatty deposits on the artery walls cracks or ruptures.

Recognizing the symptoms of a heart attack

Different people experience the symptoms of a heart attack in different ways. However, typical symptoms include some or all of the following:

- ✔ A heavy chest pain or tightness, usually experienced in the front of the chest, beneath the sternum and often radiating to the left arm, left shoulder, or jaw

- ✔ Shortness of breath

- ✔ Nausea

- ✔ Sweating

- ✔ Clamminess, cool skin, pallor

- ✔ A feeling of general weakness or tiredness

In an individual who has angina, symptoms may be particularly difficult to differentiate from the chest discomfort of angina. However, when a heart attack is occurring, chest discomfort usually is more severe and may occur while the individual is at rest or less active than usual.

The signs of a heart attack often are subtle, particularly with individuals who have diabetes. Diabetics may not have the classic symptoms of chest, shoulder, or arm discomfort. Chest pain experienced by many women likewise may not present the classic symptoms.

 When you think you're having a heart attack, call 911 and get to a hospital where therapy can be initiated to save your heart muscle from dying. New clot-busting medicines, as well as procedures such as angioplasty, often can dissolve a clot that causes the heart attack, open the blood vessel, and save some or all of the heart muscle at risk. Although some of the heart muscle usually dies during a heart attack, the remaining heart muscle continues to function and often can compensate, to a very large degree, for the heart muscle that has died.

Beating out of sync: Arrythmia

Cardiac arrhythmias, also called *cardiac dysrhythmias*, are irregularities or abnormalities in the beating of the heart. Arrhythmias are surprisingly common. They can arise in a wide variety of settings and can range from totally insignificant to life-threatening. In fact, if everyone were hooked up to a 24-hour, continuous electrocardiogram, you'd find that everyone experiences a few extra heartbeats and a few skipped heartbeats. Technically, all these extra and skipped heartbeats are cardiac arrhythmias. Yet for the vast majority, these minor irregularities carry absolutely no health consequences. More severe cardiac arrhythmias, however, can be deadly.

Looking at what causes arrhythmia

The cardiac electrical system is an exquisite grouping of cells and fibers that uses electrical impulses to tell the heart when to contract. When anything disturbs or interrupts the normal functioning of the heart's electrical system, problems with cardiac rhythm result. A variety of underlying conditions, which often are interrelated, can cause cardiac rhythm problems. These include problems related to the electrical system itself; congenital abnormalities (that is, problems that people are born with); underlying disease states or conditions, such as CAD, coronary valve disease or heart failure, stress, and so on; and behaviors such as using caffeine, tobacco, alcohol, and so on.

Recognizing the symptoms of cardiac arrhythmias

The symptoms of cardiac rhythm problems are as diverse as the problems themselves. They also range from inconsequential to life-threatening:

- **Palpitations:** Probably the least worrisome of symptoms, palpitations describe a variety of uncomfortable sensations of your heartbeat, such as the sensation that your heart is missing or skipping a beat. To some people, palpitations may feel like a fluttering in the chest. In and of themselves, these skipped or missed beats aren't terribly worrisome. However, when multiple skipped beats occur in succession, they can lead to serious problems.
- **A racing or pounding heart:** Although these symptoms can arise from strong emotion or exercise, if they occur while you're at rest, they may indicate a significant rhythm problem.

✔ **Lightheadedness or dizziness:** Everybody becomes lightheaded or dizzy every now and then, but if these symptoms are not one-time passing events, you need to have your doctor check out possible causes, which include heart rhythm problems.

✔ **Passing out:** Unlike fainting spells in which faintness may come on a bit gradually — with the world graying out and with your body going sweaty or clammy — fainting spells caused by rhythm problems tend to be sudden. Anyone who experiences a sudden fainting spell, or more than one episode of what seems to be an ordinary fainting spell, needs to seek medical attention to determine the underlying problem.

✔ **Cardiac collapse:** Cardiac collapse (also called *cardiac arrest*) is without a doubt a life-threatening emergency. Quick use of CPR and automated external defibrillation (AED) can double a person's chances of survival. Anyone who survives such an episode requires advanced electrical diagnostic techniques in the hands of a skilled cardiologist trained in the subspeciality of electrophysiology.

Be still my beating heart: Heart failure

Heart failure occurs when the heart no longer adequately pumps blood to the lungs and throughout the body. It usually is a slow process that takes place during a period of years. Underlying conditions, such as CAD, leakage from one of the heart valves, or various diseases of the heart muscle itself usually cause heart failure.

All forms of heart failure are serious health problems that require medical treatment. Taking care of yourself, seeing your physician regularly, and paying scrupulous attention to recommended treatments are important steps you can take to improve your chances of living longer. Fortunately, significant advances have occurred during the last several years in the medical profession's knowledge of heart failure and in the treatments that are available.

The heart initially compensates for small decreases in its ability to pump by doing the following:

✔ Enlarging (*dilatation*) to enable more blood into its pumping chambers

✔ Thickening the muscle walls (*hypertrophy*) to strengthen the pump and enable it to exert more force during its contraction to move more blood

✔ Beating faster to make up for decreased volume or power (like trying to pitch more, but smaller, pails of water on a fire)

The heart may try to compensate in these ways for years before you notice any symptoms. But when these mechanisms ultimately fail, significant heart failure occurs. By then, compensatory mechanisms often have become part of the problem.

Identifying the groups that heart failure affects most

Although heart failure is a very serious medical condition for anyone, some people tend to suffer more complications from heart failure than others, including

- **The aged:** The prevalence of heart failure most commonly increases with age. Men and women older than age 70 who have heart failure are significantly more likely to die from it than younger individuals.

- **Men:** Although men and women tend to get heart failure in comparable numbers, men tend to suffer more problems and don't survive as long after diagnosis as women. Researchers don't totally understand the reasons for the discrepancy.

- **African Americans:** Heart failure occurs more often (by about 25 percent) and is more often fatal in men and women who are African American than in white Americans. Although the reasons why heart failure is more prevalent and deadly among African Americans are unclear, at least two factors that undoubtedly contribute are the greater incidence among African Americans of hypertension and diabetes, which often underlie heart failure, and a pattern of less timely access to health care.

Recognizing the symptoms of heart failure

Because heart failure produces a lack of blood flow to vital organs (including the heart) and muscles, the typical symptoms of heart failure are shortness of breath, fatigue, edema, and coughing:

- **Shortness of breath:** The degree to which the heart's pumping ability has been compromised affects how short of breath you are. Mild heart failure causes symptoms with activity, while more severe forms are accompanied by symptoms at rest.

- **Fatigue:** Inadequate blood flow to the muscles and other tissues causes fatigue, which makes accomplishing any level of significant exertion, or even the activities of daily living, difficult.

- **Edema and coughing:** When the heart fails to pump adequately, fluid can accumulate in the feet, ankles, legs, and sometimes the abdomen, causing the swelling called *edema*. Fluid also can accumulate in the lungs, producing the congestion that gives congestive heart failure its name. For some individuals, lung congestion may result in persistent coughing or in wheezy or raspy breathing.

Taking Charge of Your Heart Health

Extensive research proves that you can do many things in your daily life to preserve and maximize the health of your heart — even if you already have heart disease. In fact, the number of deaths from heart disease declined 20 percent during the last decade — a decline largely based on lifestyle changes. Here are some things you can do:

- ✔ **Become physically active.** People who are physically active on a regular basis cut their risk of heart disease in half.

- ✔ **Stop smoking.** People who stop smoking cigarettes can return their risk of heart disease and stroke to almost normal levels within five years after stopping.

- ✔ **Lose 5 to 10 percent of your body weight.** Overweight people who lose as little as 5 to 10 percent of their body weight can substantially lower their risk of heart disease.

- ✔ **Be selective in what you eat.** Simple changes in what you eat can lower blood cholesterol.

By taking control of your heart health, you reap other benefits. One, many of the steps that benefit your heart health also improve your total health and fitness, to say nothing of your good looks. Two, the healthier your heart is, the greater the probability that you can stay active, mobile, and engaged in pursuits that interest you for a long, long time. Three, the healthier you are, the lower your health-care costs, and the more money in your pocket for fun things. Four, although keeping your heart healthy is not an iron-clad guarantee that you'll live longer, keeping your heart as healthy as possible can keep the Grim Reaper away longer. Finally, and most importantly, nothing slows you down or scares the family like a heart attack. Angina pain, angioplasty, coronary artery bypass surgery, and other common outcomes of heart disease aren't picnics in the park, either. Working for heart health and controlling heart disease can help you avoid these problems.

Understanding How the Mediterranean Diet Can Minimize Your Risk

Many key aspects of the Mediterranean diet can really help you reduce your risk, as well as the progression, of heart disease:

✔ **The focus on unsaturated heart healthy fats that help lower your LDL cholesterol and raise your HDL cholesterol, as well as reduce the risk for oxidation of cholesterol.** This oxidation is what leads to artery plaque build-up and, eventually, heart attack or stroke. In the Mediterranean diet, you swap out butter and limit red meat and full-fat dairy products in favor of olive oil, nuts, seeds, avocado, and fish — items that give you a dose of monounsaturated and polyunsaturated fats like omega-3s.

Omega-3 fatty acids from fish in particular help decrease your triglycerides, which is another type of fat in your blood that increases your risk for heart disease. In addition, omega-3 fats can reduce inflammation in your body that may cause damage to your arteries.

✔ **Reliance on primarily plant-based foods like whole grains, fruits, vegetables, nuts, seeds, and legumes.** These foods contain a plethora of antioxidants and fiber, which helps lower cholesterol and helps you maintain a healthy weight — all heart disease protectants. Some of the Mediterranean diet super foods in this category include

- Grains, like barley and quinoa

- Fruits, like figs and pomegranate

- Veggies, like eggplant and artichoke

- Nuts, like pine nuts, walnuts, and pistachios

- Beans, like garbanzo and cannellini

✔ **Enjoying red wine in moderation.** Having a glass of wine has been shown to have a positive link to heart health due to the antioxidants, like resveratrol, which protect the blood vessel lining in your heart.

You don't necessarily need to start drinking red wine if you don't already drink alcohol — no causal connection between red wine and heart disease exists — but the point is that it doesn't hurt! As long as you're able to keep your intake to the moderate level (one 5-ounce glass per day for women and two for men) and have no other reason to avoid wine, you're good to go when it comes to your heart health.

Chapter 4

High Blood Pressure and Stroke: A Lowdown Dirty Shame

• •

In This Chapter

▶ Getting the lowdown on high blood pressure

▶ Identifying different kinds of strokes and their symptoms

▶ Making changes in your diet and lifestyle to prevent hypertension and stroke

▶ The link between the Mediterranean diet and factors that put you at risk for stroke

• •

High blood pressure is a national epidemic. At least 40 million Americans have high blood pressure, yet estimates indicated that 40 percent of those who suffer from high blood pressure don't even know they have it. The fact is the older you are, the more likely you are to have high blood pressure, particularly if you are black. Until age 50, men are more likely than women to have high blood pressure. After the age of menopause, women are more likely than men to be hypertensive.

In a society where stress, obesity, and a landscape of convenience-food offerings high in sodium work against healthy blood pressure, it may be no surprise that hypertension is on the rise or that, even after receiving a bad blood-pressure report card from their doctor, some still don't do anything to treat the condition. Maybe it's because most of the effects of high blood pressure are not symptomatic. Years may pass before you suffer the consequences.

But the consequences of high blood pressure, or hypertension, are dire and include damaged blood vessels and heart disease, as well as putting you at high risk for a stroke. This chapter explains what high blood pressure is, who's at risk, and how to prevent it. Here you also find out the link between high blood pressure and stroke, and how making changes in your lifestyle today can help you ward off this silent killer or get it under control.

Understanding High Blood Pressure

Young blood vessels are quite rubbery. When the heart beats, the blood is forced into the blood vessels under pressure. Like a thick-skinned, tree-shaped balloon, the vessels stretch out and expand a little as the blood moves through them. When your heart beats, blood is forced through the vessels at the maximum pressure, called *systolic blood pressure*. Between heartbeats, the tight, rubbery girdle of the blood vessels squeezes back down on your blood and keeps it moving through your arteries. Your blood pressure never drops to zero between heartbeats because of your elastic blood vessels. The lowest pressure is called the *diastolic blood pressure*.

As you get older, atherosclerosis (a build-up of plaque on the blood vessel lining) and age make your blood vessels less elastic, and your heart has to beat harder to keep the average pressure up, resulting in a higher systolic pressure and a lower diastolic pressure.

High blood pressure is sometimes called the silent killer. You can have high blood pressure for years before you have any sign of problems. As the heart strains to push the blood at high pressure through arteries, it enlarges, and the arteries start to show signs of wear. Although you can have atherosclerosis without having high blood pressure, atherosclerosis is usually much worse and gets worse faster when accompanied by high blood pressure. After several years of untreated high blood pressure, you may notice some changes:

✔ You may suffer from headaches and dizzy spells, or you may have more frequent nosebleeds.

✔ As the atherosclerosis worsens, you may develop poor circulation in your feet.

✔ High blood pressure is also the number-one risk factor for stroke, and atherosclerosis can cause stroke when it results in the formation of blood clots.

How high is too high? Defining high blood pressure

Blood pressure is recorded as two numbers: the highest (systolic) pressure during a heartbeat over the lowest (diastolic) pressure between beats. For example, your doctor may tell you that your blood pressure is 120 over 80 and write it down as 120/80. (That, by the way, would be good news for you — as this is an average and normal blood pressure reading.) The highest number, the systolic pressure, is given first, followed by the lowest pressure.

So what number is considered high blood pressure? Well, various levels of blood-pressure readings set off different alarms:

- **Pre-hypertensive:** If your blood pressure is higher than 120/80 but lower than 140/90, then you are said to be pre-hypertensive and likely to develop hypertension if you don't take measures to stave it off. National guidelines recommend that you walk more, lose weight, and reduce sodium in your diet.

- **Bad and really bad:** If your blood pressure is higher than 140/90 but lower than 160/100, you have Stage 1 high blood pressure (bad). If your blood pressure is higher than 160/100, you have Stage 2 high blood pressure (really bad).

Knowing the risk factors

High blood pressure isn't the result of a single cause. Some circumstances you can't control — your age or your family history, for example. Others may require lifestyle changes or medical solutions. In any event, you'll benefit by knowing the range of conditions that may lead to high blood pressure:

- **Family history:** If you have high blood pressure, chances are pretty good that someone else in your family does, as well. If you don't have high blood pressure, and a family member does, then regardless of your age, it's important for you to check your blood pressure now and keep a close watch on it through the years. It is also good motivation to start exercising and keeping your weight under control now, actions that can help delay the onset of high blood pressure and all its problems.

- **African Americans:** African Americans as a group have a very high rate of high blood pressure. It is estimated that about 36 percent of African Americans have high blood pressure compared to 25 percent of white Americans. African Americans have approximately 50 percent more strokes than white Americans. The reasons for these differences are not known. African Americans have a higher prevalence of other risk factors, including diabetes and obesity, as well.

- **Diet and lifestyle:** Time and again, studies support that losing weight reduces blood pressure. In addition to losing weight, certain dietary factors can impact your blood pressure:

  - **Adding unhealthy sodium through table salt:** Table salt can raise blood pressure. Salt that you eat goes into your bloodstream and is excreted by your kidneys. When the concentration of salt increases in your blood, water is drawn into the blood from other tissues to dilute the salt until your kidneys have time to excrete it. The extra blood volume and extra work for the kidneys increase your blood pressure. Restricting salt may help lower your blood pressure.

- **Neglecting potassium and calcium in the diet:** Diets high in potassium promote better health and may result in lower blood pressure. Good sources of potassium are fruits such as cantaloupe, bananas, apricots, and oranges, as well as dairy products, lean meats, and dried legumes. Calcium can also help reduce your blood pressure. Key sources of calcium are dairy products. You can also find calcium in sardines, certain grains and legumes, and even vegetables such as spinach, broccoli, and celery.

- **Drinking too much alcohol:** Those who have one drink of alcohol per day have a reduced risk of stroke and heart attack. (That doesn't mean that if you don't drink you should start — it's never been shown in a clinical trial that adding one glass of alcohol per day will help those who drink less.) However, more than two to three drinks of alcohol per day can add to your risk of high blood pressure.

✔ **Kidney problems:** Kidneys play a major role in controlling your blood pressure by controlling the volume of blood and the amount of sodium and potassium in the blood. Any disease of the kidneys may affect blood pressure.

Identifying Kinds of Strokes

Stroke is the third most common cause of death in the United States, and the number-one cause of serious disability. One year after the most common kind of stroke, approximately 30 percent of those afflicted will have died, and another 30 percent will have a moderate to severe disability.

But the news is not all bad. Of those who experience the most common type of stroke, approximately 40 percent are left with only a mild disability or no disability one year later. And each year more people survive and recover from stroke as medical research continues to advance effective treatment. Today, recovery with improvement is the rule rather than the exception.

Clearly, the more you know about stroke — its symptoms, causes, risks, and prevention — the better your chances of living a full and productive life with or, better yet, without stroke.

A friend of mine, a cardiologist, once told me that neurologists make stroke too complicated with their jargon and classification. He said he just thinks of stroke like wine: There's red wine and white wine — and red stroke and white stroke. Basically, some strokes are caused by broken blood vessels — which results in blood in the brain or brain area (thus, the red); other strokes are caused by the blockage of vessels to the brain, so no blood gets there (hence, white).

I liked his use of the color-coding and have found that when I talk to patients and their families, this explanation helps them better understand the cause of the stroke and what is happening in the brain. So in the following sections, I classify the major types of stroke into these two general categories, based on whether they are caused by bleeding (red) or blockage (white).

White strokes

White strokes — technically called *ischemic strokes* or *acute ischemic strokes* (AIS) — stop the flow of blood. White strokes are the most common type of stroke, representing four out of five strokes. In almost every white stroke, a blood clot forms and blocks blood flow to a part of the brain. The result is a painless loss of brain function. Sometimes, the incident has little or no impact on a person's life; in other cases, it causes severe incapacitating disability. Most white strokes result in some kind of life-changing disability.

Factors leading to white strokes

Most of the factors that lead to forming blood clots can be related in one way or another to things you do — or don't do — that increase your chances of having a white stroke. Here are a few of key risk factors:

▸ **Having high blood pressure:** As explained earlier, hypertension is a disease that causes your blood pressure to be higher than it should be, even when you are relaxed and rested. High blood pressure quadruples your chances of having a stroke compared to people your same age who don't have high blood pressure. High blood pressure injures the lining of your blood vessels, leading to a clot, which can result in a stroke. Usually the stroke is a white (ischemic) stroke. High blood pressure is also a major risk for red strokes. Sometimes it causes a weak-walled artery to burst and bleed into the brain — a red stroke (see the later section "Red strokes").

▸ **Having atherosclerosis:** The most common sign of blood-vessel damage is atherosclerosis, the condition in which plaque forms because of high blood pressure and high fat content in your blood. The roughness makes it more likely that blood inside your arteries will form clots that can block arteries in the brain or break up into smaller pieces that are carried downstream to lodge in small brain arteries. Sometimes blood clots can break off and flow downstream to form a blockage somewhere else, called an *embolism*. Figure 4-1 shows atherosclerosis, blood clots, and embolism.

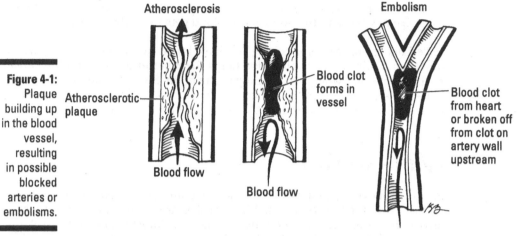

Figure 4-1:
Plaque building up in the blood vessel, resulting in possible blocked arteries or embolisms.

✔ **Smoking tobacco:** The chemicals that get into your bloodstream when you smoke tobacco irritate the lining of the blood vessels and make atherosclerosis worse. Smoking more than doubles your risk of heart attack and stroke. Smoking also increases your blood pressure.

✔ **Experiencing atrial fibrillation:** The heart is designed to pump at a steady pace in order to maintain a strong enough pressure and keep the blood flowing smoothly. The contraction of the different chambers of the heart needs to be carefully synchronized. Otherwise, the blood doesn't flow smoothly. The biggest risk factor in developing atrial fibrilation is hypertension. Head to Chapter 3 to find out more about how the heart works.

Transient strokes

White ischemic strokes may last just a couple of minutes and then clear completely. If the blood clot breaks up right away, the stroke is transient — so fleeting that no permanent tissue death occurred. These transient strokes are officially called *transient ischemic attacks*. Try to say that ten times fast. Doctors abbreviate it as TIA.

You can have more than one transient ischemic stroke. As the number of these small strokes add up, your brain can just slow down generally, and you can suffer from dementia, as each small stroke erodes away more of your brain. Small white ischemic stroke dementia is often called *vascular dementia* or *vascular cognitive impairment*. This is the death of the brain by a thousand cuts.

Red strokes

Red strokes are the opposite of white strokes. White strokes are caused by blood clots in the brain arteries, but red strokes are caused by bleeding of the brain arteries. The two types of red stroke are differentiated by where the bleeding starts:

- **Brain hemorrhage:** When you experience a brain hemorrhage, or *intra-cerebral hemorrhage* (ICH), the bleeding is within the brain itself. Brain hemorrhage produces the same signs and symptoms as a white stroke: paralysis of the face, arm, or leg on one side of the body; difficulty speaking or understanding speech; loss of sensation on part of one side of the body; dizziness; and clumsiness in the use of the arms or legs. However, a red stroke caused by brain hemorrhage often continues to get worse as the minutes and hours pass, eventually progressing to coma in many cases. A typical white stroke, on the other hand, stays the same or even improves on its own during the first few hours, and coma occurs much less often.

  Brain hemorrhages are more often fatal and cause more severe disability than the more common white ischemic stroke. The chances of someone dying in the first few days after a brain hemorrhage are about 40 percent — double the rate for white strokes, which is about 20 percent. This is primarily because of the catastrophic consequences of brain swelling that accompanies brain hemorrhage.

- **Subarachnoid hemorrhage:** In this type of stroke, bleeding occurs just outside the brain but still inside the skull. The most common cause in this case is an aneurysm, a peanut or marble-sized bubble or pouch that forms at the Y-junctions of a brain-bound artery (see Figure 4-2). An aneurysm has a tough, thin, rubbery wall and may actually be present for years before it starts causing trouble. Some never do cause trouble. But aneurysms may get larger as time passes and, as they do, they are more likely to burst. The result can be devastating, as high-pressure blood from larger brain arteries floods into the space around the brain. If you aren't killed immediately, you have to survive weeks of recovery as your body tries to clean up the resulting mess. Further injury to your brain and rebleeding are likely unless you get immediate medical attention.

This type of red subarachnoid hemorrhage stroke is usually accompanied by severe headache. Many people also fall unconscious when the stroke first hits. The pain and loss of consciousness are both strong warnings that something serious is happening.

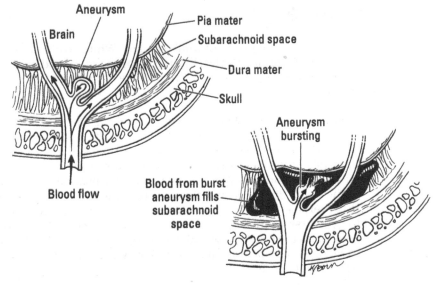

Figure 4-2:
Aneurysms
cause
bleeding in
the space
surrounding
the brain.

High blood pressure — particularly longstanding high blood pressure — is the leading cause of brain hemorrhages, being responsible for nearly half of the incidences. Over the years, high blood pressure, particularly if aggravated by diabetes, wears out and weakens the walls of small blood vessels deep inside the brain. These vessels are connected directly to high-pressure mainline arteries to the brain. They are exposed to greater stresses than other small blood vessels in the brain. After years of strain, the blood vessels develop dilapidated, patched, and repatched walls. In some places, the vessels are so weak that they form tiny *blebs* (little blisters) that can easily break under high pressure.

Blebs are little blisters on the walls of blood vessels, about the size of the head of a pin. These tiny blebs are also called *microaneurysms*, but don't confuse them with the much larger berry aneurysms that cause subarachnoid hemorrhage.

How the brain reacts to blood

The brain hates blood that isn't where it is supposed to be. And when blood gets outside of brain blood vessels, by whatever means, the brain reacts strongly. Although eventually the bleeding stops on its own as the clotting process kicks in, the repercussions can be extremely destructive. Here are just some of the challenges.

The brain swells and becomes deformed: Blood gushing from an artery into the substance of the brain makes it swell up just like any bruise under the skin or in a muscle. The extra blood alone causes the brain to swell. But the reaction also causes white blood cells to release special chemicals to respond to the blood. More white blood cells are drawn to the area. The blood vessels in the surrounding area begin to leak fluid around the blood clot. Injured brain cells also leak fluid into the substance of the brain. The result is that the brain swells even more as it reacts to the release of blood within the brain.

The problem with all this swelling is that the brain is trapped inside the skull. If the brain swells, then something else has to shrink. For a while, this can be the clear fluid around the brain and in brain ventricles. But if the brain continues to swell, something else has to give. As bleeding continues to increase the size of the brain inside the skull, the pressure in the skull goes up. It's as if the brain is pushing against the skull and all the holes in it. As the brain pushes out, the heart has a harder time pushing the blood into the skull. If the pressure gets too high, the heart will fail to push enough blood into the brain to sustain brain function.

This is a total disaster. First, the brain shuts down, leading to unconsciousness. Then before too many minutes, the brain starts to die from lack of blood flow. Sometimes there is so much blood and swelling in the brain that nothing works. Within a few minutes or hours, death occurs. Fortunately, in most cases, either the pressure doesn't get so high that blood flow stops, or the pressure inside the skull can be controlled so that blood flow continues.

The swelling from the bleeding happens on just one side of the brain, but the imbalance in pressure squeezes against the side of the brain that is not bleeding. The brain is flexible only to a certain extent. The spinal cord and nerves at the base of the brain still have to exit from the holes in the skull. They can stretch a little, but they pull back on the brain as it is deformed by the pressure. The brain can actually push part of itself down into the space in the neck where the spinal cord usually is.

There are a few really tight places where vital brain structures that keep a person alive and breathing are squeezed so hard that the nerve cells are crushed and torn. The victim loses consciousness, but this time because of actual physical injury to the brain. Injuries to the base of the brain are not easy to fix, and they are the most common cause of death for patients with brain hemorrhage.

You lose consciousness: You fall unconscious because the vital structures in the brain fail to respond to stimuli that would ordinarily keep you alert. There are different degrees of unconsciousness, but in the deepest levels of coma, the brain is not able to keep the lungs breathing.

Preventing more red strokes

Someone lucky enough to get out of the hospital after a brain hemorrhage needs to take action to prevent more strokes. A red stroke puts you at increased risk of white strokes. In addition to following all your doctor's orders to the letter (taking and monitoring any medications you're proscribed), you must also take these preventative measures:

- **Treat your blood pressure:** It's your first priority. Remember, longstanding high blood pressure causes nearly half of all brain hemorrhages. This means check your blood pressure regularly, see the doctor more often, take medication if appropriate, and make lifestyle changes (diet and exercise) as necessary.

- **Manage blood lipids, diabetes, and heart disease:** High blood pressure is intimately connected to other blood-related conditions, including high cholesterol, diabetes, and heart disease. You can read more about diabetes in Chapter 5 and heart disease in Chapter 3. Being healthy may mean giving up favorite pastimes and taking more pills than you want to. Tough luck. Work hard to live long.

Time is critical for people having a stroke. The earlier you get to the hospital, the better your chances.

Paying Attention to Signs of Stroke

Stroke is sometimes called a brain attack. Just as a heart attack threatens your heart, a stroke threatens your brain. In truth, most stroke is like a heart attack: It's a problem with blood vessels, and time is really important. However, heart attack is a little easier to recognize. First of all, the pain tells you something is wrong — and it is usually near your heart. Most strokes are painless, and the symptoms, a paralyzed arm or leg for instance, are not obviously related to the brain.

Whatever the cause, during a stroke, part of your brain may be deprived of blood and life-giving oxygen. When that happens, it doesn't take long for your brain to suffer. Typically, your brain will begin to shut down in less than a minute, and you will show signs of stroke.

The 50 professional groups forming the Brain Attack Coalition describe the signs of stroke as follows:

- Sudden numbness or weakness of face, arm, or leg, especially on one side of the body

- Sudden confusion, trouble speaking or understanding speech

- Sudden trouble seeing in one or both eyes

✔ Sudden trouble walking, dizziness, loss of balance or coordination

✔ Sudden severe headache with no known cause

A stroke doesn't hurt (except if a headache accompanies it), and its most obvious effects are far from the brain where the problem is located — factors that make it difficult for you to recognize that the reason your hand looks funny and doesn't move when you want is because there's something wrong in your head. In fact, most people who have a stroke don't know what's happening to them. Most people who see someone who's had a stroke don't know what's happening, either.

The end result is that a lot of people don't recognize they are having a stroke and can't use the opportunities they have to get into the hospital quickly and be treated.

Taking Steps to a Healthier You

The fact is neither you nor I nor your doctor knows for certain whether a stroke is in your future. It's not really possible to predict with any certainty exactly who will suffer a stroke. To some extent, having a stroke is a matter of bad luck.

What is known is that certain characteristics place you at a greater risk for stroke. You are more prone to suffer a stroke if you have high blood pressure, smoke cigarettes, and/or have heart disease, diabetes, or high blood cholesterol levels. Researchers have identified a number of indicators that can help predict the likelihood of stroke. Some you can influence; others you can't.

Unfortunately, you may be carrying some genetic, hereditary, gender, or age baggage that you simply can't change, such as

✔ You've already had a stroke.

✔ You are 65 or older.

✔ You are African American.

✔ You are Hispanic.

✔ Stroke runs in your family.

✔ You are a man.

✔ You have diabetes.

So you can't change your age, your sex, your past, or your forebears' genetic makeup. But there are plenty of other ways to make changes in your life that will significantly reduce your risk of stroke. Following are some of the steps you can take to improve your outlook for a stroke-free future.

Treating high blood pressure

For people who have never had a stroke, treating blood pressure cuts the risk of stroke nearly in half. In older patients, treating people with systolic high blood pressure reduces the chances of dementia by half. If you've had a stroke, the chances you will have a second one are reduced by 30 percent if you treat your high blood pressure.

There isn't much good data on how much to lower the blood pressure. Most evidence shows that the lower, the better. However, in the majority of studies, the average reduction in blood pressure has been only about ten points.

If there isn't a treatable cause of high blood pressure (hyperthyroidism, for example), there are two basic ways to lower your blood pressure:

- ✔ Diet and exercise
- ✔ Medication

Because they don't treat the cause of the high blood pressure, these treatments have to be continued every day. Because the dosage or types of medicine may change over time, you must work closely with your doctor. Regular and frequent monitoring of your blood pressure helps ensure that your treatment program is working. If you are taking medicine for blood pressure, you should still exercise and eat a healthy diet.

Your efforts will be well worth it in preventing not just heart attack and stroke, but a number of other life-threatening health conditions, listed in Table 4-1.

Table 4-1	The Effects of High Blood Pressure
Effect	*Risk*
Hardening of arteries (arteriosclerosis)	Heart attack, stroke
Bulges in blood vessels (aneurysms)	Bleeding due to ruptured aneurysms
Enlarged heart	Heart failure, heart transplant
Injury to kidney blood vessels	Kidney failure and dialysis
Burst arteries in retina of eye	Vision loss, blindness

Managing your weight and diet

If you're overweight, consume an unhealthy menu of high-sodium and high-fat foods, and you avoid regular exercise, you may be able to lower your blood pressure and your risk of stroke by making some positive lifestyle changes. Even if you are recovering from a stroke, you can follow these recommendations:

- ✔ Exercise enough to make you breathe faster.
- ✔ Get your weight under control.
- ✔ Eat more fruits high in potassium (such as cantaloupe, bananas, apricots, and oranges).
- ✔ Restrict your sodium intake by cutting back on table salt.
- ✔ Consume low-fat dairy products to increase your calcium.
- ✔ Enjoy alcohol up to one or two drinks per day but avoid more.
- ✔ Avoid cold tablets and diet drugs that have warnings about high blood pressure.

A healthy diet also helps you lower "bad" cholesterol and raise "good" cholesterol. If diet alone doesn't do the trick, talk with your doctor about cholesterol-lowering medications.

Other things you can do

In addition to lowering your blood pressure and managing your weight through diet and exercise, you can also decrease your risks if you stop smoking.

The evidence is overwhelming that, when you stop smoking, you can reduce your odds for having stroke. After a year or two, your chances of stroke are reduced to the same as if you had never smoked. For information on how to quit smoking, go online to www.dummies.com/extras/mediterraneandiet.

Discovering Diet Components That Reduce Your Risk

Specific research has shown that the Mediterranean diet is inversely related to your diastolic and systolic blood pressure. That means you can keep your blood pressure within normal limits — and, therefore, lower your risk for stroke — by following classic Mediterranean habits like the following:

✔ **Making olive oil one of your primary fat sources in lieu of butter or other saturated fats.** In fact, consuming olive oil every day (3 to 4 tablespoons) has been correlated with a 50 percent decrease in the need for blood pressure medications. The magic ingredient may be polyphenols, which are antioxidants that help the lining of blood vessels relax, effectively lowering blood pressure.

✔ **Consuming minimally processed, real foods like fresh fruits, vegetables, nuts, seeds, and whole grains.** Because the Mediterranean people stick to foods that are grown locally, they get more of the good stuff such as antioxidants, fiber, and potassium without additives that contain sodium, which facilitates increases in blood pressure.

Potassium is a major mineral in the body that helps regulate muscle contraction and normal heart functioning. Mediterranean favorites containing plenty of potassium include mandarin oranges, avocados, sweet potatoes, white beans, and fish, like salmon.

✔ **Being active.** Although not exactly diet-related, the Mediterranean people get their fill of physical activity. Biking and walking are more ingrained in their culture than mass-transit. The American Heart Association recommends getting about 30 minutes per day of activity to keep the heart strong and pumping blood efficiently.

If you don't exercise regularly, take it slow. You don't need to vigorously workout to benefit from what activity has to offer. Start by going for walks around the neighborhood or taking a fun exercise class to keep it interesting so that you'll stay engaged! Go online to www.dummies.com/extras/mediterraneandiet for suggestions on how to get moving.

Chapter 5

Digging into Facts about Diabetes

. . . .

In This Chapter

▶ Distinguishing between type 1 and type 2 diabetes

▶ Identifying the complications caused by diabetes

▶ Noting the link between diet, exercise, and managing or preventing diabetes

▶ Looking at the benefits the Mediterranean diet offers those with diabetes

. . . .

The Greeks and Romans knew about diabetes. The way they tested for the condition was — prepare yourself — by tasting people's urine. In this way, the Romans discovered that the urine of certain people was *mellitus*, the Latin word for sweet. (They got their honey from the island of Malta, which they called Mellita.) In addition, the Greeks noticed that when people with sweet urine drank, the fluids came out in the urine almost as fast as they went in the mouth, like a siphon. The Greek word for siphon is *diabetes*. Thus we have the origins of the modern name for the disease, diabetes mellitus.

This chapter provides a general overview of diabetes: its symptoms, the populations at risk, and ways to avoid it or minimize its complications. As you read, you'll discover that, beyond the factors you can't control, like genetics, that may put you at risk for diabetes, there are other factors you can control: namely your diet and activity level — which is where the Mediterranean diet comes in.

Defining Diabetes and Its Types

The standard definition of diabetes mellitus is excessive glucose in a blood sample. The cause of the excessive glucose can be that the body doesn't produce sufficient amounts of insulin (as in type 1 diabetes) or it doesn't use the insulin efficiently (as in type 2 diabetes).

Of course, diabetes doesn't suddenly appear one day without previous notification from your body. For a period of time, which may last up to ten years, you may not quite achieve the criteria for a diagnosis of diabetes but not be quite normal either. During this time, you have what's called prediabetes.

Understanding type 1 diabetes

Type 1 diabetes is an autoimmune disease, meaning that your body is unkind enough to react against — and in this case, destroy — a vital part of itself, namely the insulin-producing beta (B) cells of the pancreas. People who get type 1 diabetes more often have certain abnormal characteristics on their genetic material, their chromosomes, that are not present in people who don't get type 1 diabetes. Another essential factor in predicting whether you will develop type 1 diabetes is your exposure to something in the environment, most likely a virus that diminishes your ability to produce insulin, which quickly creates the diabetic condition in your body.

Type 1 diabetes used to be called *juvenile diabetes* because it occurs most frequently in children. However, so many cases are found in adults that doctors don't use the term juvenile any more.

Following are some of the major signs and symptoms of type 1 diabetes:

- ✔ Frequent urination
- ✔ Increased thirst
- ✔ Weight loss, despite an increase in hunger
- ✔ Weakness

To prevent complications from type 1 diabetes — including eye, kidney, and nerve disease — the most important thing you can do is control your blood glucose level to keep it as close to normal as possible. If you already suffer from such complications, improving your blood glucose control slows the progression of the complications. You achieve this control through medications and adherence to a healthy diet. To find out much more on the subject of type 1 diabetes, read *Type 1 Diabetes For Dummies,* by Alan Rubin (John Wiley & Sons, Inc.).

Understanding type 2 diabetes

Unlike type 1 diabetes, type 2 diabetes isn't a condition of the autoimmune system, nor is a virus believed to trigger onset. In addition, type 2 occurs gradually. Because the symptoms are so mild at first, you may not notice them, and years may pass before they become bothersome enough to spur you to consult your doctor. Recent statistics show that ten times more people worldwide have type 2 diabetes than type 1 diabetes, making type 2 much more prevalent.

Recognizing the symptoms of type 2 diabetes

Exhibiting two or more of the following signs and symptoms is a good indicator that you have type 2 diabetes:

✔ **Fatigue:** Type 2 diabetes makes you tired because your body's cells aren't getting the glucose fuel that they need. Even though your blood has plenty of insulin, your body is resistant to its actions. (See the next section, "Investigating the risk factors of type 2 diabetes" for more on insulin resistance.)

✔ **Frequent urination and thirst:** As with type 1 diabetes, you find yourself urinating more frequently than usual, which dehydrates your body and leaves you thirsty.

✔ **Blurred vision:** The lenses of your eyes swell and shrink as your blood glucose levels rise and fall. Your vision blurs because your eyes can't adjust quickly enough to these lens changes.

✔ **Slow healing of skin, gum, and urinary infections:** Your white blood cells, which help with healing and defend your body against infections, don't function correctly in the high-glucose environment present in your body when it has diabetes. Unfortunately, the bugs that cause infections thrive in the same high-glucose environment. So diabetes leaves your body especially susceptible to infections.

✔ **Genital itching:** Yeast infections also love a high-glucose environment, so diabetes is often accompanied by the itching and discomfort of yeast infections.

✔ **Numbness in the feet or legs:** You experience numbness because of a common long-term complication of diabetes called _neuropathy_. (I explain the details of neuropathy in the later section "Other diseases and conditions.") If you notice numbness and neuropathy along with the other symptoms of diabetes, you probably have had the disease for quite a while, because neuropathy takes more than five years to develop in a diabetic environment. Occasionally numbness occurs earlier when extreme elevations of the glucose happen.

✔ **Heart disease, stroke, and peripheral vascular disease:** Heart disease, stroke, and peripheral vascular disease (blockage of arteries in the legs) occur much more often in people with type 2 diabetes than in the non-diabetic population. But these complications may appear when you are merely glucose-intolerant (which I explain in the next section), before you actually have diagnosable diabetes.

A 2007 study showed that, in a group of over 15,000 people being treated for diabetes, 44 percent of people with type 2 diabetes reported not one of the symptoms above in the previous year when given a questionnaire. It is no wonder that a third of people with diabetes don't know they have it!

Investigating the risk factors of type 2 diabetes

Doctors know quite a bit about the risk factors for type 2 diabetes:

- **Family history of the disease:** Type 2 diabetes runs in families. Usually, people with type 2 diabetes can find a relative who has had the disease. In studies of identical twins, when one twin has type 2 diabetes, the likelihood that it will develop in the other twin is nearly 100 percent.

- **Insulin resistance:** People with type 2 diabetes have plenty of insulin in their bodies (unlike people with type 1 diabetes), but their bodies respond to the insulin in abnormal ways. Being insulin resistant means that your body resists the normal, healthy functioning of insulin. This resistance, combined with other factors such as weight gain, a sedentary lifestyle, certain medications, and aging, create a situation in which your pancreas can't keep up with your insulin demands, and you develop pre-diabetes, followed by diabetes.

- **Being overweight or obese:** The number of people who have type 2 diabetes is on the rise, and one reason is an increase in the incidence of obesity. If you're obese, you are considerably more likely to acquire type 2 diabetes than you would be if you maintained your ideal weight. The most important environmental factors that turn a genetic predisposition to type 2 diabetes into a clinical disease include

    - **High body-mass index:** The body-mass index (BMI) is the way that doctors look at weight in relation to height. BMI is a better indicator of a healthy weight than just weight alone. For instructions on calculating your BMI, head to Chapter 6.

    - **Physical inactivity:** Physical inactivity has a high association with diabetes, as evidenced in study after study. One, which did not include any obese people, showed that the occurrence of diabetes was greatest for people who don't exercise.

    - **Central distribution of fat:** When people with diabetes become fat, they tend to carry the extra weight as centrally distributed fat, also known as visceral fat, which stays around your midsection. Visceral fat seems to cause more insulin resistance than fat in other areas, and it is also correlated with the occurrence of coronary artery disease (refer to Chapter 3). You can check your visceral fat by measuring your waistline.

    Fortunately, visceral fat happens to be the type of fat that is relatively easy to lose when you diet. If you have a lot of visceral fat, losing just 5 to 10 percent of your weight may very dramatically reduce your chance of diabetes or a heart attack.

• **Low intake of dietary fiber:** Dietary fiber seems to be protective against diabetes because it slows down the rate at which glucose enters the bloodstream. Populations with a high prevalence of diabetes tend to eat a diet that is low in fiber.

People often think that eating excessive amounts of sugar causes type 2 diabetes, but simply eating lots of sugar actually has nothing to do with the onset of the disease. However, doing so can make you fat, which is a huge risk factor in developing the disease. Eating too much protein or fat does the same thing.

✔ **Age:** Your chances of getting type 2 diabetes increase as you get older. Although most people with type 2 diabetes are over the age of 40, more and more cases are occurring in children and young adults.

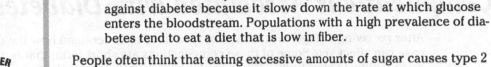

Getting a wake-up call from prediabetes

Prediabetes exists when the body's blood glucose level is higher than normal but not high enough to meet the standard definition of diabetes mellitus. A person with prediabetes doesn't usually develop eye disease, kidney disease, or nerve damage (all potential complications of diabetes, discussed in later sections of this chapter). However, a person with prediabetes has a much greater risk of developing heart disease and brain attacks than someone with entirely normal blood glucose levels.

Despite how many people have prediabetes, most of them don't know it. People at risk for prediabetes have one or more of the following risk factors:

✔ Belonging to a high-risk ethnic group: African American, Hispanic, Asian, or Native American

✔ Being overweight

✔ Having high blood pressure

✔ Having low "good" (HDL) cholesterol

✔ Having high levels of triglycerides

✔ Having a family history of diabetes

✔ Having diabetes during a pregnancy or giving birth to a baby weighing more than 9 pounds

Diagnosing prediabetes can be the best thing that ever happened to a person! It could be the wake-up call that motivates you to make crucial lifestyle changes, especially in diet and exercise, which have been shown to prevent the onset of diabetes in people with prediabetes.

Complications Associated with Diabetes

After receiving a diagnosis of diabetes, you need to understand how the disease can affect you. Some of these complications are short term; that is, they arise rapidly in your body. Others are long term, in that they take ten or more years to develop. In either case, these complications can affect your ability to function normally.

Hypoglycemia (low blood glucose)

Your body doesn't function well when you have too little glucose in your blood. Your brain needs glucose to run the rest of your body, as well as to function intellectually. Your muscles need the energy that glucose provides in much the same way that your car needs gasoline. In the worst scenarios, hypoglycemia can lead to coma and even death.

You can control blood sugar levels (which you want to stay in a normal range — neither too high or too low) through medication (insulin shots), diet, and exercise.

Controlling blood sugar levels is like trying to balance a teeter-totter. The goal is to keep the levels from spiking or plummeting. The kinds and amount of food you eat, as well as how much time passes between eating, impact how steady your blood sugar level is. Similarly, exercise impacts blood glucose levels because when you're active, your body burns energy in the form of sugar, thus lowering blood glucose levels. People who exercise regularly require much less medication and generally can manage their diabetes more easily than nonexercisers can. For those with diabetes, figuring out the right combination is the key to maintaining an acceptable blood sugar level.

Kidney disease

With kidney disease (also known as nephropathy), your kidneys lose the ability to filter your blood of waste. When that happens, you must either use artificial means, called *dialysis*, to cleanse your blood or receive a new working donor kidney via a transplant. Other than uncontrolled blood sugar levels, factors that increase your chances of developing kidney disease include

- **High blood pressure (hypertension):** This factor may be almost as important as the glucose level. Refer to Chapter 4 for information on high blood pressure.

✔ **Factors of inheritance:** Certain families and ethnic groups have a higher incidence of diabetic nephropathy.

✔ **Abnormal blood fats:** Research shows that elevated levels of certain cholesterol-containing fats promote kidney disease.

To prevent kidney disease or significantly slow it down after it begins, control your blood glucose, control your blood pressure, control the blood fats (that is, lower you bad cholesterol, raise your good cholesterol, and lower triglycerides), and take any blood pressure medication your doctor prescribes.

Eye disease

The eyes are the second major organ of the body affected by diabetes over the long term. Common eye problems in diabetics include cataracts (opaque areas of the lens that block vision), glaucoma (high pressure inside the eye that damages the optic nerve), and diabetic retinopathy (caused by high levels of blood glucose over time that can lead to blindness).

Patients with severe diabetic retinopathy are at increased risk for heart attacks. An article in *Diabetes Care* in July 2007 strongly confirmed this relationship. People with diabetic retinopathy are twice as likely to have a heart attack as people with diabetes who don't have retinopathy. If they have a heart attack, it's three times as likely to be fatal.

If you have diabetes, you must get an annual eye examination by an ophthalmologist or optometrist to preserve your vision. Doctors who are not ophthalmologists or optometrists diagnose retinopathy correctly only 50 percent of the time, while ophthalmologists and optometrists are correct more than 90 percent of the time. You need to get an eye examination as soon as you are diagnosed with type 2 diabetes or five years after the diagnosis of type 1 diabetes, and you need to be rechecked every year after that.

Heart disease

In the last three decades, the number of deaths due to heart disease has fallen dramatically, thanks to all kinds of new treatments as well as improved diets. However, the tremendous increase in the number of type 2 diabetes patients predicted for the next few decades may reverse this trend. In this section, you find out about the special problems that diabetes brings to the heart. (To find out more about heart disease, refer to Chapter 3.)

Controlling the blood glucose, the blood fats, and the blood pressure early in the disease help to lessen or prevent coronary artery disease.

Coronary artery disease

Coronary artery disease (CAD) is the term for the progressive closure of the arteries, which supply blood to the heart muscle. If CAD is severe, it can lead to heart attack. In fact, CAD is the most common reason for death in patients with type 2 diabetes. Women with type 2 diabetes are at increased risk for CAD compared to men.

If a heart attack occurs, the risk of death is much greater for the person with diabetes. More than half of all people with diabetes die of heart attacks. If people without diabetes have heart attacks, they die 15 percent of the time, but people with diabetes die 40 percent of the time. The death rate is worse for people with diabetes who poorly controlled their glucose before the heart attack.

The following risk factors promote CAD in type 2 patients:

- Increased production of insulin, caused by insulin resistance.
- Obesity and having fat concentrated in the waist area

  Studies indicate that body-mass index is not a good predictor of heart attacks and death in obese diabetic patients. The waist in inches divided by the height in inches is the best predictor (a waist-to-height ratio under 0.5 is considered healthy), followed by the waist circumference (less than or equal to 40 inches in men and 35 inches in women is lower risk), followed by the waist-to-hip ratio (under 0.9 in men and 0.8 in women is healthy).

- Hypertension (high blood pressure)
- Elevated "bad" (LDL) cholesterol and decreased "good" (HDL) cholesterol
- Sitting time, especially long stretches of inactivity, such as watching television for a long time

Previous studies show that red wine is good for your heart. Recent studies suggest that white wine has substances that are heart healthy as well, and both have alcohol, which is healthy in moderate amounts (two drinks daily for men and one for women).

Metabolic syndrome

The earliest abnormality in type 2 diabetes is insulin resistance, which is found in people even before diabetes can be diagnosed. People with impaired glucose tolerance, and even 25 percent of the population with normal glucose tolerance, have evidence of insulin resistance. The condition, formerly known as *insulin resistance syndrome*, is now called *metabolic syndrome*.

Metabolic syndrome is believed to be present in one-third of all Americans. Overweight males (those with BMIs of 25 or greater) are 6 times as likely to have metabolic syndrome, and obese males (with BMIs of 30 or greater) were 32 times as likely. Interestingly and for reasons that are not yet known, people who consume diet sodas daily have been found to have an increased risk of metabolic syndrome and type 2 diabetes. In addition, the syndrome is being found in obese children and adolescents, resulting in greater danger of diabetes and an early heart attack.

Several conditions or characteristics accompany insulin resistance. Among those are

- ✔ Hypertension

- ✔ Abnormalities of blood fats (elevated levels of triglycerides and bad cholesterol and decreased levels of good cholesterol)

- ✔ Presence of *C-reactive protein*, a marker for inflammation in the body, and increased levels of *plasminogen activator inhibitor-1*, a chemical that prevents the breakdown of blood clots that form in the arteries

- ✔ Obesity and increased abdominal visceral fat

- ✔ Sedentary lifestyle

A number of treatments are available for the metabolic syndrome. If you are obese and have a sedentary lifestyle, you should correct these problems. Even a small amount of weight loss — 5 to 10 percent of your body weight — or exercise can make a major contribution toward decreasing the risk of a heart attack. An exercise training program has reversed metabolic syndrome in 30 percent of patients.

Vascular diseases

The same processes that affect the coronary arteries can affect the arteries to the brain, producing cerebrovascular disease, and the arteries to the rest of the body, producing peripheral vascular disease:

- ✔ **Peripheral vascular disease (PVD):** When arteries are clogged to parts of your body other than the heart and brain, you experience the loss of pulses in the feet; after ten years of diabetes, a third of men and women no longer feel a pulse in their feet. The most common symptom of PVD is intermittent pain or cramping in the calves, thighs, or buttocks that begins after some walking and subsides with rest. People with PVD have lower life expectancy. When PVD occurs, just as when CAD occurs, it is much worse in people with diabetes because more of their arteries are involved. The following risk factors are within your control:

- Smoking, which promotes early foot amputation
- High cholesterol
- High glucose
- High blood pressure
- Obesity

✔ **Cerebrovascular disease (CVD):** CVD is a disease of the arteries that supply the brain with oxygen and nutrients. If a temporary reduction in blood supply to the brain occurs, the person suffers from a transient ischemic attack, or TIA. This temporary loss of brain function may present itself as slurring of speech, weakness on one side of the body, or numbness. TIA may disappear after a few minutes, but it comes back again some hours to days later. If a major artery to the brain completely closes, the person suffers a stroke. For more information on strokes, refer to Chapter 4.

People with diabetes are at increased risk for CVD, and their disease tends to be worse than the disease in a person without diabetes. They can have blockage in many small blood vessels in the brain that leads to the loss of intellectual function, a symptom similar to Alzheimer's disease.

Smoking and diabetes

Smoking has a number of ill effects on people without diabetes, but the effects are even worse in people with diabetes. Among other things, smoking has the following consequences:

✔ Reducing blood flow in arteries and blocking increased flow when it is needed

✔ Increasing pain in the legs in people with CVD and in the heart in people with CAD

✔ Increasing *atheromatous plaques,* the changes in arteries in the heart and other areas (like the brain and the legs) that precede closing of the blood vessels

✔ Increasing clustering of *platelets,* the blood elements that form a plug or clot that blocks the artery

✔ Increasing blood pressure, which also worsens atheromatous plaques

These problems don't even take into account the effects of smoking on the lungs, the bladder, and the rest of the body. For tips on how to quit smoking, visit www.dummies.com/extras/mediterraneandiet.

Other diseases and conditions

People with diabetes can suffer from a number of other conditions, such as the following:

- **Nerve disease (neuropathy):** Sixty percent of people with diabetes have some abnormality of the nervous system. These patients usually don't realize it, because the disease doesn't have any early symptoms. These patients usually have poor glucose control, smoke, and are over age 40. Nerve disease is found most often in the people who have had diabetes the longest. Diabetic neuropathy often leads to foot infections, foot ulcerations, and amputation — complications that are all entirely preventable.

- **Disorders of movement (mononeuropathy):** Disorders of movement occur when you lose motor nerves that carry the impulses to muscles to make those muscles move. When you lose those nerves, you lose the ability to move or use those muscles. These disorders are believed to originate as a result of the sudden closing of a blood vessel supplying the nerve. The clinical picture depends on which nerve or nerves are affected. If one of the nerves to the eyeball is damaged, for example, the patient can't turn his eye to the side that nerve is on. If the nerve to the face is affected, the eyelid may droop, or the smile on one side of the face may be flat. The patient can have trouble with vision or problems with hearing. Focusing the eye may not be possible. No treatment really exists, but fortunately the disorder goes away on its own after several months.

- **Diabetic foot disease:** About 70,000 amputations occur in the United States each year, and more than half of them are done on people with diabetes. Good medical care can prevent amputations. Your doctor should look at your feet as routinely as he or she measures your weight.

- **Skin diseases:** Many conditions involving the skin are unique to diabetic people because of the treatment and complications of the disease. The most common and important skin complications include bruising; conditions, such as vitiligo and necrobiosis lipoidica, that affect skin pigmentation; acanthosis nigricans, a velvety-feeling increase in pigmentation on the back of the neck and the armpits; dry skin; fungal infections; and more.

- **Gum disease:** The gums may develop gingivitis, becoming brittle and bleeding easily. You may experience pain and bad breath, and eventually the gums may become so weakened that they cannot support your teeth.

- **Sleep apnea:** Sleep apnea is characterized by recurrent episodes, lasting 10 to 30 seconds each, of failure to breathe while asleep. In a study of over 300 patients with type 2 diabetes and obesity, over 86 percent of the patients had obstructive sleep apnea. Waist circumference was a key indicator of obstructive sleep apnea.

Using Diet and Exercise to Prevent or Help Control Diabetes

You may wonder what you have to do to prevent the complications of diabetes described in the preceding sections, and the answer is a fair amount. Diabetes management has three major aspects: monitoring glucose levels, eating a proper diet, and getting sufficient exercise.

None of these tasks is particularly easy, but when you weigh the benefits that add up to a longer, better-quality life against the loss of time and money from preventive care, the benefits of preventive care win by a landslide. The following sections provide the details, and because high blood pressure exacerbates so many of the conditions associated with diabetes, you can also find information on the importance of controlling your blood pressure, too.

Another key component of managing diabetes is taking the appropriate medication. The kind and amount of medication you take depend on whether you have type 1 or type 2 diabetes and how well you are able to control it on your own through diet and exercise. For some people, medication is a must from the get-go; for others, dietary and lifestyle changes can make the difference between needing medication and not.

Monitoring glucose levels: It's a must!

Insulin was extracted and used for the first time more than 80 years ago. Since that time, nothing has improved the life of the person with diabetes as much as the ability to measure his or her own blood glucose with a drop of blood.

Basically, two kinds of test strips are used today. Both require that glucose in a drop of your blood reacts with an enzyme. In one strip, the reaction produces a color. A meter then reads the amount of color to give a glucose reading. In the other strip, the reaction produces electrons, and a meter converts the amount of electrons into a glucose reading.

Being able to accurately measure your blood-glucose level enables you to take steps to make adjustments as needed to keep your glucose levels within the acceptable range.

Eating a proper diet

As the earlier sections in this chapter make clear, those with diabetes need to be very careful about what they eat, not only because the foods they choose have a direct impact on their blood glucose levels but also because diet plays a big part in whether they suffer from conditions — like high blood pressure and obesity — that tend to be associated with diabetes or make the diabetic complications worse.

By following a careful nutrition program, a person with diabetes can reduce the severity of the disease and reduce or prevent altogether many of the associated health complications. The following sections offer some highlights.

Consuming the right amount and right kinds of carbohydrates

Carbohydrates are the sources of energy that start with glucose, the sugar in your bloodstream that is one sugar molecule, and include substances containing many sugar molecules called *complex carbohydrates*, *starches*, *cellulose*, and *gums*. Some of the common sources of carbohydrate are bread, potatoes, grains, cereals, and rice. Fiber is the part of the carbohydrate that is not digestible and, therefore, adds no calories. Fiber is found in most fruits, grains, and vegetables.

All carbohydrates are not alike in the degree to which they raise the blood glucose. To address that fact, a measurement called the *glycemic index* was created. People with diabetes should select carbohydrates with low GI levels. A glycemic index of 70 or more is high, 56 to 69 is medium, and 55 or less is low. Foods that are excellent sources of carbohydrate but have a low GI include legumes, such as peas or beans; pasta; and grains, like barley, parboiled rice (rice that is partially boiled in the husk, making it nutritionally similar to brown rice), bulgur, and whole-grain breads.

Switching to low GI carbohydrates can be very beneficial for controlling glucose. Table 5-1 lists simple substitutions people with diabetes can make in their diets. As an added bonus, many of the low GI foods also contain a lot of fiber, which helps to reduce the blood glucose.

Table 5-1	Simple Diet Substitutions
High-GI Food	*Low-GI Food*
White bread	Whole-grain bread
Processed breakfast cereal	Unrefined cereals like oats and processed low-GI cereals
Plain cookies and crackers	Cookies made with dried fruits or whole grains like oats
Cakes and muffins	Cakes and muffins made with fruit or whole grains like oats
Tropical fruits, like bananas	Temperate-climate fruits, like apples and plums
Potatoes	Pasta and legumes
White rice	Basmati and other low-GI rice

Clinical studies have shown that, all other things being equal, the people with the highest GI diet most often develop diabetes. After diabetes is present, patients who eat the lowest GI carbohydrates have the lowest levels of blood glucose. The other thing that happens when low GI food is incorporated into a diet is that the levels of triglycerides and "bad" (LDL) cholesterol fall in both type 1 and type 2 diabetes.

Portioning proteins

Excluding vegetable sources of protein like soybeans, legumes, nuts, and seeds, protein in your diet is usually the muscle of other animals, such as chicken, turkey, beef, or lamb. Your choice of protein is very important because some is very high in fat, and some is practically fat-free. Table 5-2 lists the various sources of protein, categorized by leanness.

Table 5-2	Protein Sources		
Very Lean	*Lean*	*Medium-fat*	*High-fat*
Skinless white-meat chicken or turkey	Lean beef, lean pork, lean lamb, or lean veal	Most beef products; regular pork, lamb, or veal	Pork spare-ribs or pork sausage
Flounder, halibut, or tuna canned in water	Dark-meat chicken without skin or white-meat chicken with skin	Dark-meat chicken with skin or fried chicken	Bacon
Lobster, shrimp, or clams	Sardines, salmon, or tuna canned in oil	Fried fish	Processed sandwich meats
Fat-free cheese	Other meats or cheeses with 3 grams of fat per ounce	Cheeses with 5 grams of fat per ounce, such as feta and mozzarella	Regular cheeses like cheddar or Monterey Jack

You can probably guess that low-fat and high-fat proteins have a huge difference in calories. An ounce of skinless white-meat chicken contains about 40 calories, whereas an ounce of pork spareribs has 100 calories.

Many authorities recommend less protein in the diet because protein has a damaging effect on the kidneys. Several studies have shown this to be the case, but a very large study in the *Annals of Internal Medicine* in March 2003 came to a different conclusion. It showed that high-protein diets caused increasing damage in kidneys that already had some damage but not in normal kidneys. The jury remains out on this question of lower versus higher protein diets.

Filling the fat requirement

People with type 2 diabetes have to be very aware of the fats in their diet. Everyone agrees that you should eat no more than 30 percent of your diet as fats. (Currently, the U.S. population eats 36 percent of its diet as fats.)

Some fats are more dangerous in their tendency to promote coronary artery disease than others. These fats should make up less of the dietary fat than the safer fats. Pay particular attention to foods that increase triglycerides, which lead to the production of small, dense LDL particles that are connected to coronary artery disease. Triglycerides come in several forms:

✔ Saturated fat is the kind of fat that usually comes from animal sources. The streaks of fat in a steak are saturated fat. Butter is made up of saturated fat. Bacon, cream, and cream cheese are other examples. Vegetable sources of saturated fat include coconut, palm, and palm-kernel oils. Eating a lot of saturated fat increases your blood cholesterol level.

Saturated fats should make up less than a third of the 30 percent of your total daily calories that come from fat.

✔ Trans fatty acid is produced when polyunsaturated fat (which I describe in the next bullet) is heated and hydrogen is bubbled through it. Fully hydrogenated, it becomes solid fat; partially hydrogenated, it has a consistency like butter and can be used in butter's place.

Trans fatty acids may contribute more to the development of heart disease than saturated fats. Keep them out of your diet! Some examples of foods high in trans fats are some cake mixes and dried soup mixes, many fast foods and frozen foods, baked goods like donuts and cookies, potato chips, crackers, breakfast cereals (even some with seemingly health-conscious names), candies, and whipped toppings. The government now requires food labels to list trans fats, so read those labels! Fortunately, food manufacturers are increasingly removing trans fats from their products.

✔ Unsaturated fat comes from vegetable sources. It comes in these forms: monounsaturated fat, which does not raise cholesterol and is found in foods like avocado, olive and canola oils, and nuts like almonds and peanuts; and polyunsaturated fat, which does not raise cholesterol but reduces good cholesterol and is found in soft fats and oils such as corn oil and mayonnaise.

Keep your dietary cholesterol, which is a key culprit in the development of coronary artery disease, peripheral vascular disease, and cerebrovascular disease, under 300 milligrams per day.

Getting sufficient exercise

Exercise plays a role in maintaining acceptable glucose levels, maintaining a healthy weight, and providing protection against a variety of conditions, like high blood pressure, that tend to plague those with diabetes.

In the *Standards of Medical Care in Diabetes 2012,* the American Diabetes Association makes the following recommendations:

- ✔ People with diabetes should perform at least 150 minutes each week of moderate-intensity aerobic physical activity (50 to 70 percent of maximum heart rate), spread over at least three days per week, with no more than two consecutive days without exercise.

  A great exercise is walking. Go online to www.dummies.com/extras/ mediterraneandiet to find a strategy that gets you walking 10,000 steps a day.

- ✔ In the absence of a medical reason not to, people with type 2 diabetes should perform resistance training at least twice per week.

Although exercise cannot replace medication for someone with type 1 diabetes, its benefits are crucial for patients with both types of diabetes. The major benefit of exercise for both types of diabetes is to prevent macrovascular disease (heart attack, stroke, or diminished blood flow to the legs). Macrovascular disease affects everyone, whether they have diabetes or not, but it's particularly severe in people with diabetes.

Exercise prevents macrovascular disease in numerous ways:

- ✔ Helps with weight loss, which is especially important in type 2 diabetes. Increased physical activity prevents weight gain as you age and weight regain if you diet. Exercise, even without weight loss, reduces the risk of diabetes.

- ✔ Lowers bad cholesterol and triglycerides, and raises good cholesterol.

- ✔ Lowers blood pressure.

  All the complications of diabetes are made worse by an elevation in blood pressure, especially diabetic kidney disease but also eye disease, heart disease, nerve disease, peripheral vascular disease, and cerebral arterial disease.

- ✔ Lowers stress levels.

- ✔ Reduces the need for insulin or drugs.

- ✔ Reduces C-reactive protein, a cause of heart and blood vessel disease in diabetes.

Possibilities for future prevention of diabetes

Researchers have performed many valuable studies on the prevention of type 2 diabetes. The results of these studies suggest that you can prevent diabetes, but probably only by making major lifestyle changes and sticking to them over a long period of time. Here are some important conclusions based on prevention research:

✔ Exercising regularly may delay the onset of diabetes.

✔ Maintaining a proper diet can delay the onset of diabetes and slow the complications that may occur.

✔ Controlling both your blood pressure and your blood glucose has substantial benefits for preventing the complications of diabetes.

The results of the Diabetes Prevention Program, a study of more than 3,000 people, were published in the *New England Journal of Medicine* in February 2002. They clearly showed that diet and exercise are effective in preventing type 2 diabetes. Participants who successfully modified their diet and exercise routines reduced their chances of developing type 2 diabetes by 58 percent. They generally did 30 minutes of moderate exercise (like walking) every day and lost between 5 and 7 percent of their body weight during the three-year study period.

Components of the Mediterranean Diet That Help You Avoid or Control Diabetes

Diabetes is a global health problem. Type 2 diabetes is especially prevalent where obesity is common. In 2008, more than 1.5 billion people worldwide were overweight, and 500 million people were obese. Currently 366 million people have diabetes. Diabetes is most concentrated in areas where large food supplies allow people to eat more calories than they need. Several different types of diabetes exist; the type 2 diabetes, the kind usually associated with obesity, is far more prevalent than the other types.

One very interesting study traced people of Japanese ancestry who moved from Japan to Hawaii to the United States mainland. Here's what researchers found: In Japan, where people customarily maintain a normal weight, the people tended to have a very low incidence of diabetes. As they moved to Hawaii, the incidence of diabetes began to rise along with their average weight. On the U.S. mainland, where food is most available, these Japanese had the highest rate of diabetes of all.

In general, as people migrate to areas of the world consuming a Western diet, not only do the number of calories they consume change, but the composition of their diets also changes. Before they migrate, they tend to consume a low-fat, high-fiber diet. After they reach their destination, they adopt the local diet, which tends to be higher in fat and lower in fiber. The carbohydrates in the new diet are from high-energy foods, which don't tend to be filling and which, in turn, promote more caloric intake.

The Mediterranean diet doesn't only help with diabetes because of its ability to promote weight loss and help you maintain a healthy weight. Studies also show that people who eat a Mediterranean-based diet have a decreased risk of diabetes even without losing weight or changing their activity levels. One study published in *Diabetes Care* in 2010 found a 52 percent decrease in diabetes incidence from changes in diet alone! Another one found that people were about 20 percent less likely to need diabetes medication after following a Mediterranean diet when compared to a traditional low-fat diet.

So what else besides weight loss is the diet impacting?

- ✔ **Improved blood glucose control.** By choosing more whole grains and fiber-full carbohydrates instead of refined carbohydrates, you improve your blood glucose levels and are less likely to have spikes. Spikes and drops in blood glucose impact the release of insulin, as well as your cravings. The Mediterranean diet emphasizes whole grains like quinoa, bulgur, and barley, and fruit for dessert. Although refined carbohydrates are included in the Mediterranean repertoire, they are consumed in smaller portions and less frequently than in the Western diet. That way, blood glucose is more controlled, and you're less likely to succumb to food cravings, which helps keep your portions in check.

- ✔ **Reduced insulin resistance.** The prevalence of olive oil, specifically extra virgin olive oil, as a main source of fat can help improve insulin resistance. The monounsaturated fats within olive oil may play a role in making your cells more sensitive to insulin and more receptive to taking up glucose.

- ✔ **Reduced inflammation.** Because the Mediterranean diet is mainly plant-based, it's chockfull of foods that help reduce inflammation. On a Mediterranean diet, people seem to have lower levels of the inflammatory markers that are predictive of diabetes. (One such marker is *adiponectin,* a protein found in fat cells which plays a role in the development of insulin resistance.) The key nutrients that help reduce inflammation in the body include fiber, omega-3 and monounsaturated fatty acids, flavonoids, and carotenoids — the key components of the Mediterranean food groups: fruits, vegetables, whole grains, nuts, seeds, fatty fish, and olive oil!

I don't mean to undermine the importance of weight loss in reducing your risk of diabetes. In fact, if you are overweight, it's very important! The Mediterranean diet helps with weight loss because it emphasizes whole, unprocessed foods and provides nutrition to fill you up and keep you satisfied. Even if you aren't focused on weight loss per se, it's an added perk of following the Mediterranean diet. Being at a healthy weight also helps you keep your blood glucose in check and can ward off insulin resistance more effectively.

Chapter 6

Wrestling with Obesity

....

....

*I*t's a sad story, but the vast majority of folks nowadays are on the fast track to fat like a runaway freight train in a summer blockbuster movie. The saddest part isn't so much the daily discomfort and inconvenience as it's the cumulative effects of lugging around those extra lipids. That added weight can actually take years off your life and possibly plague your days with illness and disease.

So what's a person to do? The good news is that obesity-related diseases and illnesses are preventable for the vast majority of people if they just lose the excess pounds and maintain a healthy body weight. And contrary to popular assumption, very few people actually have a genetic predisposition to weight gain because of variations in hormones and metabolism. This means that you have hope, although the sooner you act, the better. The solution is simple, but it sure ain't easy sometimes.

This chapter arms you with a lot of information so you understand how your weight affects your overall health and takes you through the process of reaching your fitness goals even when they seem overwhelming (minus all the fad diets and overhyped weight-loss strategies, of course!). It also explains how following a Mediterranean diet can play a vital role in weight management.

Understanding Healthy Body Weight

Determining your "perfect" weight from a table can be difficult for the simple reason that everybody is different. Some people have bigger bone structures, more muscle mass, and/or carry weight in different areas of the body. These variations in people's frames make using any tool that categorizes someone as overweight or obese difficult.

Your ideal body weight is the eventual weight that your body adjusts to when you have a consistently healthy approach to eating and exercise. Your body wants to naturally maintain this weight based on your physiologic makeup. It may take some time to determine this number if you have weight to lose.

The most common method for determining your ideal weight is the body mass index (BMI), a mathematical calculation of a person's ideal mass (weight) based on his or her height and weight.

The BMI doesn't discriminate between muscle, fat, or bone. People who know that they're at their ideal weight based on their nutrition and other fat measurements can and should ignore the BMI; if you have a greater amount of muscle than most people, this generalized calculation isn't going to apply to you. In general, however, a person's BMI score is a relatively good tool for people between the ages of 18 and 65. It isn't accurate for pregnant women, weightlifters, competitive athletes (their extra muscle adds extra weight even though they aren't overweight), or people with various chronic illnesses (they can suffer from muscle wasting and malnutrition).

Calculating body mass

Figuring out your body mass index sounds like an exercise in quantum physics, but don't despair; plenty of online tables do the work of calculating your BMI for you, given your height and weight. However, if you're the mathematical type who wants to check your figures against the tables, you can figure out your BMI in either pounds and inches or kilograms and meters:

- **Pounds and inches:** Calculate BMI by dividing weight in pounds (lbs) by height in inches (in) squared, and multiplying by a conversion factor of 703.

    Weight (lb) ÷ [height (in)]^2 × 703

    Example: Weight = 170 lbs, Height = 6' (72")

    Calculation: [170 ÷ (72)^2] × 703 = 23.05

- **Kilograms and meters:** You can calculate the BMI using the metric system by using weight in kilograms (kg) divided by height in meters (m) squared. Most often the height is measured in centimeters, so you have to convert the centimeters (cm) to meters by dividing the height by 100.

    Weight (kg) ÷ [height (m)]^2

    Example: Weight = 70 kg, Height = 183 cm (1.83 m)

    Calculation: 70 ÷ (1.83)^2 = 20.10

Recognizing unhealthy body mass

For the most part, the higher the BMI, the higher the associated health risks. By BMI standards, people with a body mass index of 20 to 25 are within range of their ideal body weight. If your BMI goes over 25, you're creeping into the dreaded "overweight" category. Following is a breakdown of the categories of BMIs that are outside the ideal range:

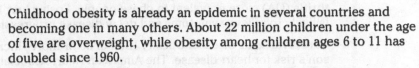

- ✔ **Overweight:** A person with a body mass index (BMI) of 25 to 29.9. Approximately 127 million adults (or 60.5 percent) in the U.S. are overweight. About 1 billion people in the world are overweight.

  Childhood obesity is already an epidemic in several countries and becoming one in many others. About 22 million children under the age of five are overweight, while obesity among children ages 6 to 11 has doubled since 1960.

- ✔ **Obese:** A person with a BMI of 30 to 39.9. About 60 million adults (or 25 percent) in the U.S. are obese, and 300 million obese adults exist worldwide. This number doesn't include children — one of the fastest growing obesity groups.

- ✔ **Morbidly obese:** A person 100 pounds over his normal weight or with a BMI of 40 or more. In the U.S., 9 million adults (or 5 percent) are morbidly obese. This group has a definite increase in obesity-related illness and mortality. The good news is that people in this BMI category can lose the weight, just like the people in the other weight categories.

The Tolls of Extra Weight

Being just "a little bit overweight" doesn't mean that you can sit back and feel safe from the serious health concerns associated with being overweight. The most important fact to take away from this chapter is that if you're even a little overweight, you are just that — over your healthy weight — and you should try to get down to a healthy weight.

The majority of researchers feel that being overweight shares the same health risks as being obese. It's easy, especially in today's overweight world, to ignore a little extra weight, especially if you're the thinnest one in your family or in your circle of friends. But this tendency can give you a false sense of comfort that can be dangerous to your health.

Most people aren't aware of the range of medical conditions directly associated with being overweight or obese — from the mildly unpleasant heartburn to death from stroke or heart disease. Yes, it's that serious. According to the *Journal of the American Medical Association*, obesity is the second-leading contributor to preventable death in the U.S., right after smoking. The heavier a person is, the less mobile he becomes, which then leads to a more detrimental, sedentary lifestyle. Weight gain and poor nutrition precipitate lack of exercise and becoming sedentary, which then increases risk for illness and disease — it's a vicious cycle.

Approximately 30 illnesses and diseases are linked to being overweight. The following represent only a handful of these medical conditions:

- **Arthritis:** Pain, stiffness, and loss of mobility of the hands, hips, back, and especially the knees are worse in people with a BMI of 25 or greater. The joints are put under a greater load of pressure that makes osteoarthritis (OA) more prevalent in obese people. Losing just 10 to 15 pounds is likely to relieve symptoms and delay disease progression.

- **Cardiovascular disease:** Obesity (BMI of 30 or more) increases a person's risk for heart disease. The American Heart Association recognizes obesity as a major risk factor for heart attack. Weight loss helps blood lipid levels by lowering triglycerides and LDL (lousy) cholesterol and increasing HDL (healthy) cholesterol.

- **Diabetes (type 2, adult onset, non-insulin-dependent diabetes):** The number of type 2 diabetics keeps increasing annually. As many as 90 percent of individuals with type 2 diabetes are reported to be overweight or obese. If you're overweight, losing as little as 5 percent of your body weight can reduce your high blood sugar.

- **High blood pressure:** More than 75 percent of high blood pressure cases are reported to be directly attributed to being overweight.

- **Sleep apnea:** Between 60 and 70 percent of people who have sleep apnea (they temporarily stop breathing while they sleep) are obese. Obesity is the largest risk factor for developing this condition.

- **Strokes:** People with a BMI over 25 increase their risk of ischemic stroke (from fatty deposits that obstruct blood vessels to the brain). Being overweight or obese is associated with high cholesterol leading to atherosclerosis (narrowing of the arteries). Atherosclerosis is a direct risk factor for strokes.

In addition to those direct links, consider the following facts:

- National Cancer Institute experts concluded that obesity is associated with cancers of the colon, breast (postmenopausal), endometrium (the lining of the uterus), kidney, and esophagus.

- Forty-two percent of those diagnosed with breast and colon cancers are obese.

- Of all gallbladder surgery, 30 percent is related to obesity.

The good news is that being over your ideal weight isn't a disease with no cure, but rather a condition with multiple cures. Keep reading and see that achieving a healthy weight is something that's very attainable.

The government started recording life expectancy in 1900. The current obesity epidemic may well lead to the first downward turn in those numbers in the future. *The New England Journal of Medicine* already projects that obesity will decrease life expectancy by close to a year; other researchers see life expectancy numbers dropping by as much as five years in the near future.

Assessing Your Current Level of Health

No one ever said losing weight was easy. Okay, maybe some people say that, but they're usually people who have never had any weight to lose! Listing what you have to do to lose weight is easy; finding the right combination of what works for you can end up being a lifelong pursuit. It's an all-out tug of war, with your body fighting to hang on to every pound. The more you fight with your body, the more your body's going to win.

So, where do you begin? This section tells you how to get ready for the battle of the bulge — check in with your physician before checking in at the gym. You also find out what you need to know about your own health before you can tailor those workouts to be beneficial and safe. Finally, this section also covers your current weight and your goal weight to give you a good idea of the road ahead.

Evaluating your fitness level

Before beginning an exercise routine, ask yourself, "What's my baseline fitness level?" Translation: How active are you? Are you overweight? Do you exercise now? How many minutes a week do you exercise? Do you lift weights or do aerobic exercise? These questions give you, your doctor, and/or your personal trainer an idea of what your basic fitness level is.

Getting the green light from your primary physician

Checking with a doctor before starting an exercise routine or weight-loss program is much more than just a legal disclaimer, so don't let this advice go in one ear and out the other. Some conditions and symptoms may require medical attention prior to jumping into exercise, just to make sure that your new exercise plan is right for you. This is a safety precaution; always err on the side of caution and see your doctor if you have any concerns.

If you're starting an exercise routine that consists of walking or light weights and you have no medical conditions or complaints, you probably don't need medical clearance. If you're not sure whether you need to see a doctor before starting a new or restarting an old exercise program, go through this health questionnaire. A "yes" answer to any of these questions means that you should consult a medical doctor first:

- Are you over the age of 40?

- Are you overweight?

- Do you smoke?

- Have you been sedentary for a long time?

- Are you starting an exercise program that involves more than walking or light weights?

- Has a doctor told you that you have a heart murmur?

- Has anyone in your family died of heart disease prior to the age of 55?

- Do you have a high risk of coronary heart disease or stroke?

- Do you have any medical conditions, such as high cholesterol, diabetes, high blood pressure, or kidney disease?

- Do your ankles swell?

- Have you experienced severe pain in your leg muscles while walking?

- Do you get short of breath more than usual when you're performing routine tasks?

- Have you fainted or do you have dizziness?

- Have you experienced any abnormal heartbeats or chest pain either at rest or when exerting yourself?

Relax — there aren't many situations where your doctor tells you that you can't exercise in some fashion. People with heart disease used to be discouraged from exercising, but studies show that, in many cases, exercise under medical supervision is helpful for patients with stable heart disease. Remember, though, that it's often difficult for a doctor to predict health problems that may arise as the result of an exercise program, so if you are at risk for any health problems, be aware of any related symptoms while you exercise.

After getting the green light to exercise, it's time to put your plan into action (before you change your mind).

Crunching your body composition numbers

The BMI determines body mass — not fat percentage. For the percentages, you need a body composition analysis, which splits your body weight into individual components: most commonly, lean mass and fat mass.

Lean body mass is actually the weight of your tissues other than fat; muscles, bones, organs, and fluids of your body, of which 50 to 60 percent is water. Body fat mass is the percent of the body that is fat and is an important number that sets the mark for the rest of the body analysis. To figure your body composition, you measure the percent of fat mass, and then subtract that number from 100 to get the percentage of lean mass.

The ideal fat percentages for men and women differ. Men have a normal range of 8 to 25 percent body fat while women should be in the range of 18 to 32 percent body fat. All the testing measures in the following sections are inexpensive options to discover more about your body makeup.

Measuring waist circumference

All fat isn't created equal — one type of fat has more potential health concerns than the other. People with central obesity (think beer bellies), or fat that is predominantly found in the abdomen (visceral fat, which is fat packed around the organs in the abdomen), tend to have more health-related illnesses than those with mostly subcutaneous fat, which is the type of fat just under the skin and is largely located in the thighs and buttocks. (See Figure 6-1 for an illustration.)

The ideal waist measurement for women is less than 35 inches. For men, an ideal waist is less than 40 inches. Go over 35 inches for women or 40 for men, and you increase your risks for health problems — regardless of height. If your BMI is in the normal range but your waist measurement isn't, go with your gut, literally — your waistline overrules your BMI on this one. (*Note:* This measurement isn't your belt size, but the circumference around the top of your hips.)

Assessing overall fat and muscle percentages

A body composition analysis uses specific tools that calculate the percentage of body fat and muscle mass to determine a person's ideal weight. By far the most common tool is the simple skinfold caliper, a quick, cheap, and noninvasive device that most trained health or fitness professionals can use. It usually requires taking three measurements at different sites of the body (triceps, abdomen, and upper thigh) by pinching and measuring subcutaneous body fat at several points and then plugging these numbers into a formula that calculates body fat. Because the tool is manual, it may have a 3 to 5 percent error in measurement — the measurement can be affected by the skill level of the professional using the tool, and the measurement isn't accurate for obese patients. (See Figure 6-2 for an illustration of how the skinfold caliper is used.)

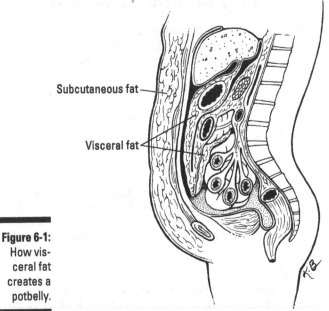

Subcutaneous fat

Visceral fat

Figure 6-1:
How vis-
ceral fat
creates a
potbelly.

Illustration by Kathryn Born, MA

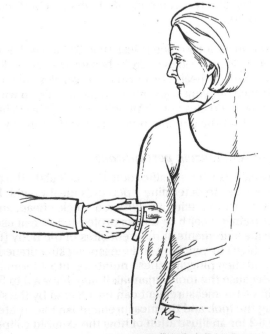

Figure 6-2:
A skinfold
caliper is
the simplest
method for
calculating
your per-
centage of
body fat.

Illustration by Kathryn Born, MA

Custom-Designing Your Plan with Balance in Mind

With so many opportunities to supersize, and so many unhealthy food choices prominently displayed in grocery stores, making healthy food choices and sticking to them in the long run are harder than ever. It can be easy to yo-yo between starving yourself and stuffing yourself, instead of settling comfortably in the middle (which is where you really need to be). After all, whether you spend your life worrying about your weight or neglecting it entirely, you're not living healthfully.

The simple math is this: The cause of weight gain is eating more calories than you burn. Your body gains 1 pound for every 3,500 calories it doesn't use. People who exercise daily throughout their lives maintain their ideal body weight more easily than those who don't.

Counting calories for weight loss

Eating right is the best thing you can do for weight loss. Exercise is always important, but what you eat and how much is much more important for maintaining a healthy weight. If you exercise heavily for one hour every day of the week but don't change your diet, you may not lose any weight.

You can find a lot of dieting options out there, and most of them center on getting a good balance of protein and carbohydrates. Drop your calories down to between 1,200 and 1,800 calories based on exercise intensity and body size. The goal is to decrease your calorie intake by 500 calories below the minimum calories that you utilize in a day and then you lose 1 pound per week. This reduction in calories results in weight loss in most cases and 1 to 2 pounds per week is a healthy weight loss rate.

Creating a safe and effective exercise program

After a doctor clears you to exercise, and you have some physical assessments done, you should be able to compile a personalized exercise program to follow. If you don't have the help of a personal trainer, set up a program based on your level of experience.

Covering the bases: The components of a complete routine

A common misconception for people who are just starting a routine is to focus only on cardio. But in that case, your body burns the energy stored in your muscles first and burns fat only as a last resort. A body transformation occurs most efficiently by simultaneously gaining muscle through strength training and losing fat through aerobics and diet. It's like a tricycle — all three wheels have to turn at the same time.

Keep these components in mind as you build your personalized program:

- ✔ **Aerobic training:** Activities like walking, swimming, and biking are all good for the lungs and heart.

  Go online to www.dummies.com/extras/mediterraneandiet to find a plan that will get you walking 10,000 steps a day.

- ✔ **Strength training:** This is the only activity that slows muscle and bone loss while it promotes weight loss.

  Your body needs energy to sustain muscle mass because muscle cells are metabolically demanding (high-maintenance); for every pound of muscle you add, your body burns 30 to 50 more calories a day even at rest. How's that for a great bargain! (And those burned calories are more likely to come from fat reserves, which is really the whole point if your goal is to lose body fat.)

- ✔ **Flexibility training:** To maintain good muscle health and reduce injury, incorporate flexibility training through stretching, yoga, and Pilates. These activities not only feel good but also increase the range of motion of your joints.

In order for your routine to work and be effective, it has to be something you want to do and take full responsibility for. So, while you decide what kind of workout you want (weight training and aerobics), where you're going to get it (at the gym or on the bike trail), and which days of the week to devote to which activity (Monday: gym, Wednesday: rollerblade in the park, Thursday: swimming), personalize and work with your routine until it's comfortable. Then, of course, you start working out. Many people are wonderful at putting plans together — and terrible at implementing them! The best exercise plan in the world won't do a thing for you unless you actually do it.

People who have been sedentary for long periods (at least 6 to 12 months) may be at a higher risk for injury because muscle tone is weak, flexibility is limited, and balance is shaky. *Note:* Although most people consider walking the first step in becoming active, starting with strength training may be safer and more beneficial for people with limitations in their mobility (joint disease) or aerobic capacities (advanced lung disease).

Factoring in your personality and lifestyle

When starting an exercise routine, you need to first evaluate your personality and lifestyle. If you create a routine that you don't enjoy, can't afford, or can't squeeze in, chances are good that you won't stick with it. Ask yourself the following questions:

✔ **What motivates me?** Motivation (or the lack of it) has the power to start and stop a routine as fast as you can spit the word out. So find activities that you enjoy. You may be someone who just won't do aerobic activities like running or biking, but can play basketball or soccer for hours. Go for it! Sporting activities are great sources of exercise, and joining a league locks you into a schedule. If paying for a membership gets you to commit to the gym because you want to get your money's worth, buy a gym membership. You can get motivated, but sometimes you have to be creative.

✔ **Can I stick to my guns all on my own, or do I need the support of a group?** If you need the support of a group, consider a taking an exercise class, joining a support group, engaging in a planned weight-loss program, or finding a workout partner or personal trainer.

✔ **What type of programs meet my health needs and interest me?** Carefully consider what keeps you coming back for more.

✔ **What resources are available to me, and how much money am I willing to spend?** You can find an exercise program for any budget. Remember that allocating funds for your health is an investment that can reduce medical visits, medications, and time off work. It could be the best money you spend!

✔ **What time of day is best for me to work out?** There's really no perfect time of day that maximizes your workouts. Some researchers have tried to designate a particular workout time based on hormones and body rhythms, but no solid data is available. Some environmental restrictions, such as heat, cold, or rain, may make certain times of the day safer (and make you less likely to cancel). Bottom line? The best time of the day is the time that's consistently available to you with the least interruptions.

Getting the goods

You don't need to purchase expensive gym equipment to get a good workout. Sporting goods stores as well as major discount department stores have all sorts of products for at-home users or people who want companion pieces for their exercise classes. Here's a list of some basic equipment to get you started:

✔ **Handheld weights:** Hand weights (also known as dumbbells) are a must-have for any do-it-yourselfer. They range in increments from 1 to 10 pounds, and then go up to 12 and 15 pounds.

If you're adding hand weights to your daily walk, go light because there's a risk of joint inflammation and injury, especially if you use heavier weights and don't do adequate warm-up. If you're doing bicep curls, try a few reps in the store. When your muscles fatigue at 15 repetitions, you've found a good starting weight.

✔ **Resistance bands:** Resistance bands are long tubes that look like rubber jump ropes with handles. These bands are easy to use at any age or fitness level and offer your muscles a full range-of-motion workout.

✔ **Exercise stability balls:** Who would've thought that sitting on a big, round ball would be a workout? Seems like mere child's play until you try to balance yourself and realize that your body is using micro muscles you forgot you had!

✔ **Floor mat:** A closed-cell (nonabsorbent to wick away moisture) foam mat that's at least ⅜ of an inch thick is great to avoid slipping and to provide comfort and support.

✔ **Workout DVD:** You can find an endless variety of workouts for every age, lifestyle, and fitness level. Try one from your local movie rental store or your public library before you buy it.

✔ **Good quality shoes:** A comfortable and supportive pair of sneakers with rubber soles and good arch support is essential.

From trial to style: Making a (good) habit of it

Whatever the reason for starting an exercise routine or a healthy-eating regimen, you need to have even better ones for keeping the fire burning. Too often, the smallest hurdle (a broken fingernail, a mild headache, or a friend saying, "Let's go to lunch!") can put out that fire. To help avoid this pitfall, keep these suggestions in mind:

✔ **Make exercise a priority.** Set a time in your schedule for exercise and stick to it.

✔ **Practice saying no.** When friends and family try to interfere with your workout plans or suggest that "one little cookie won't hurt," say no.

✔ **Implement a system of checks and balances.** Trying to lose weight requires sacrifices every day — but those sacrifices are balanced by the rewards. You have to get yourself ready by recognizing the difficult situations that make it hard to make those sacrifices. For instance, don't have candy in the house if you love candy. Out of sight, (hopefully!) out of mind.

Sacrifice is important, but torture is unnecessary. Make sure that you have checks in place to increase your chances of success. If you like coffee in the morning, have the coffee, but also drink more water. If you like to have a beer in the evening, switch to a light beer. If you want to have dessert on occasion, work out three days a week to balance out those calories. To succeed in the fitness world, finding balance is essential. When you establish balance, it becomes habit and a new lifestyle.

Sometimes, despite their best efforts, people encounter the slump of discouragement and frustration, especially when they've tried to lose weight more than once, only to gain it back. To bounce back from those self-defeating thoughts and feelings, refocus with the following methods:

- Focus on the process instead of the end result.
- Focus on what went well today (or this week) and the successes.
- Use visualization and imagery techniques to focus on yourself at your goal weight, participating in an enjoyable activity.
- Focus on physical activity as an opportunity to do something enjoyable.
- Put away the scale for a while and focus on making lasting lifestyle changes. As a result, the weight will come off.

Finding the rewards at the end of your rainbow of sacrifices is easy. Every time you reach one of your goals, reward yourself. Every positive action deserves a pat on the back. Get some new clothes or take a mini-trip. And make sure that you set reasonable goals, because the rewards are that much more valuable.

Succeeding at the Hardest Part: Maintaining Your Healthy Weight!

Healthy eating is the biggest component of weight loss. Exercise definitely helps, and is most important for burning off extra calories from those situations when you stray from your normal dietary habits such as vacations, parties, or just dessert after a good meal out. Weight maintenance, on the other hand, is the result of successfully incorporating good nutrition and routine daily exercise into your lifestyle.

The key to keeping off weight

Many people can lose weight, but they gain the weight back quickly. Becoming a yo-yo dieter, one who loses weight and gains it back just to try to lose it again in what turns into a vicious cycle, isn't healthy and can become expensive if you have to buy new clothes or expensive diets and diet supplements.

Weight maintenance comes down to a few things:

- Making consistently smart food choices
- Staying committed to an exercise routine that's enjoyable and rewarding

- ✔ Maintaining plenty of balance and patience
- ✔ Weighing yourself weekly; what you don't know can hurt you
- ✔ Refusing to let "just a few little pounds" creep back up on you without taking immediate action
- ✔ Setting goals that work for you, not for someone else

Living life somewhere in the middle is apt to lead to more positive and long-lasting results than living in the extremes. And people who are able to successfully keep their weight down are the ones who have figured out how to make balanced choices. This isn't to say that you'll never eat another double fudge chocolate sundae — only that you've figure out how to make it part of your balanced choices.

Overcoming all-too-common obstacles to a healthy weight

There's nothing terribly complicated about living a healthy, life-prolonging lifestyle. So why are more people falling prey to partially preventable diseases every year? This section explores what we think are the biggest reasons behind the staggering numbers of preventable death. Take these pointers to heart, so you can recognize any that may be present in your own life and make the modifications to effectively enhance the quality of your life, both now and in the future, no matter what your age.

Short-sighted thinking

We're going to let you in on a little secret: everyone is mortal. Despite this being common knowledge, few people think about the inevitability of their own death and the things they can do to prevent it from happening prematurely. If they did, there would be far fewer accidents of every type, no one would ever break their hip falling off a ladder they shouldn't have been on in the first place, and cigarette sales would plummet.

The idea that death can be postponed leads to thinking that "tomorrow" is a good time to start a dietary overhaul, an ambitious new exercise regimen, and, of course, tomorrow is the best time to quit smoking and drinking.

We're not advocating that you get out the sackcloth and ashes and carry a sign that states "The End is Near," but a little realism can go a long way toward a new way of living that can literally save lives — at least for a few more years.

Confusing what feels good with what is good

Making healthy food choices can have a major impact on health. Most people know some of the fundamental eating habits that should be avoided such as eating fried foods and high sugar content snacks. Those same people also know that fruits and vegetables are good for you. Then why are so many people unable to make the decision to eat the way they know they should?

Could it be that some people's inability to stop eating poorly is an addiction, similar to addictions to tobacco and alcohol? More likely, it's the cavalier attitude many people have about their health that keeps them eating poorly, until they're slapped in the face with the reality of poor health. You may have heard the saying "cancer is the cure for smoking." Well, you would think diabetes and heart disease would be the cure for obesity . . . but sadly, they often aren't.

Moving to healthy eating habits is difficult. Eating what's good for you just doesn't feel as good as eating what's bad for you, in many cases. It's not that you can't ever eat a fast-food meal again — you can. You can't, however, eat fast food or packaged food all or even most of the time and stay healthy.

The desire for a quick (and easy) fix

Given a choice, most people will take the quick fix over hard work every time. Lose 25 pounds in a week, guaranteed? Sign me up! Quit smoking overnight? Here's my money! Build a beautiful body in only two minutes a day — and you don't even have to stand up? That's for me!

It's human nature to want something for nothing, but when it comes to living healthfully, you have to put in the time and effort — hours in the gym, self-control in the grocery store, and discipline in your lifestyle choices. And make no mistake, it takes time and effort to eat healthier foods, exercise, and maintain a focused, balanced low-stress lifestyle. You have to give up things — horribly unhealthy foods that taste so wonderful as well as time you feel short on anyway — to get yourself in a positive routine.

Seeing How the Mediterranean Diet Helps with Weight Management

One of the beautiful side effects of following a Mediterranean diet is weight loss or healthy weight maintenance. Consider it a "side effect" because this type of diet is not your typical restrictive meal plan you may hear about in the media. It's not a quick fix (that doesn't exist, by the way), nor will you feel deprived when eating like the people in the Mediterranean do. Instead, you'll reap all the benefits of nutritious foods and enjoy your meals and your lifestyle, all while reducing your risk for obesity and promoting, as research also shows, a smaller waistline. Here's why the Mediterranean diet helps with weight loss and healthy-weight maintenance:

- ✔ **It focuses on real foods.** When you swap out less processed and packaged foods and swap in whole, nutritious, real foods in your diet, you get better nutrition without the junk. The Mediterranean diet is a plant-based diet with a strong focus on fruits, veggies, nuts, seeds — the good stuff! These foods are chockfull of fiber, vitamins, and minerals, all of which help keep you satisfied on fewer calories than the processed stuff has and are correlated with lower weight. That way, you're better able to keep your portions and calories in check. At the same time, you're ditching fast foods, foods high in sugar, and high fat meats and dairy, which contribute to obesity.

- ✔ **It focuses on healthy fats.** The use of olive oil as the main source of fat, paired with omega-3 fatty acids from fish, nuts, and seeds, has been shown to have a protective effect on weight gain. Fat, in general, ensures you feel satisfied from the foods you're eating instead of feeling deprived. And that deprived feeling is the main reason why many "diets" fail in the first place.

- ✔ **It focuses on activity.** Although not technically part of the diet, activity is a huge part of the Mediterranean lifestyle. Instead of mass transit, the people of the Mediterranean walk and cycle more to get to where they need to be. Any amount of activity you do is better than nothing, but aim to be moderately active at least 30 minutes per day. Doing so not only helps your weight but also helps you avoid or reduce abdominal fat, which is correlated with a higher risk for disease. Getting active also clears your head and reduces stress, which may make it easier for you to stick to healthy habits all around!

Chapter 7

The Topic of Cancer

Cancer. It's the nightmare diagnosis that most people fear more than any other. And who can blame them? Not too long ago, the diagnosis itself was akin to a death sentence. Cancer drugs — even early ones — were miracles of modern science, but they, too, exacted a cost. Fast-forward to today. Many cancers are treatable, but a cancer diagnosis, even for a highly treatable form of cancer, is still enough to frighten you and shake up your world.

Nevertheless, more than ever before, the words *cancer* and *death* do not necessarily belong in the same sentence. Each day brings news of improvements in screening tests and in treatments. And, happily, survival rates for cancer are at an all-time high in the United States. And more and more research reaffirms how a healthy lifestyle — including diet and exercise — can reduce your chances of developing cancer.

The American Cancer Society, which crunches data from the National Cancer Institute (NCI, www.cancer.gov), the Centers for Disease Control and Prevention (CDC, www.cdc.gov), the North American Association of Central Cancer Registries (NAACCR, www.naaccr.org), and the National Center for Health Statistics (NCHS, www.cdc.gov/nchs), projects that 1,660,290 new cancer diagnoses and 580,350 cancer deaths will occur in 2013 — despite the fact that the overall cancer rates and deaths have declined slightly.

Demystifying the "C" Word

Cancer is a disease — more accurately, a group of diseases — and every person's body carries within it the possibility of developing cancer. Cancer also is a disease on the run. Due to the development of more sophisticated detection methods and improved courses of treatment, the number of people surviving cancer in the United States has more than tripled over the past 30 years — so says the National Cancer Institute and the Centers for Disease Control and Prevention.

Understanding how cancer develops

Just what is cancer? The disease originates at the cellular level. Cells, you may recall from biology class, grow and divide as necessary to ensure that you have all the cells you need to maintain a healthy body. As you read this, some 10 million of your cells are busy dividing. This is normal.

Usually, cell division is an orderly process, with cells growing, maturing, and then dying off as new cells take their place. Sometimes, for reasons not entirely understood, this routine is interrupted. A single cell that has undergone a mutation — either a spontaneous change as a result of a natural incident or one resulting from exposure to a *carcinogen,* or cancer-causing agent — begins to reproduce and keeps at it, without stopping. These new cells, which never reach maturity, form a growth or mass of tissue, and that mass is a tumor.

Tumors come in two types: benign and malignant:

- ✔ **Benign tumors:** Generally, benign tumors stay put and do not spread to other parts of the body. If a benign tumor is surgically removed, it usually does not come back.

- ✔ **Malignant tumors:** These tumors contain abnormal cells that continue to divide. Sometimes these cancerous cells invade tissue or nearby organs and try to destroy the healthy cells. Sometimes they enter the bloodstream or the lymphatic system, and when that happens, the cancer cells can spread to sites in the body distant from the site at which the cancer originated. If it spreads, the cancer is termed *metastatic* — more about this topic in the upcoming section "Differentiating among tumors."

What causes cancer?

About 10 percent of the people who get cancer get it because of abnormalities in their genes. Lots of research is under way to try to pinpoint these abnormalities and find ways to deal with them even before cancer develops. But no one yet knows exactly why particular cells become cancerous while others don't.

Demystifying the "C" word

The origin of the word *cancer* is as comical as the connotation is scary. Studying cancers of the breast, uterus, stomach, and skin in the fifth century BCE, Hippocrates observed that a cancerous tumor (shown here) has a hard center with "claw-like projections" — a shape similar to a common crustacean. The good doctor named the disease *karkinos* or *karkinoma*, the Greek word for crab, giving us *carcinoma*. The Latin version of the Greek word is *cancer*.

Hippocrates is, of course, the same Greek physician who gave his name to that famous oath that physicians take upon graduation from medical school.

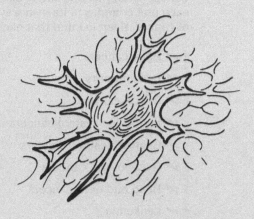

Illustration by Kathryn Born, MA

Plenty of other factors can also take the blame. Some, considered identified risk factors because studies have conclusively proven the link between them and developing cancer, include smoking, an unhealthy diet, and unprotected exposure to the sun's rays. We talk more about these factors in the section "Considering Risk Factors," later in this chapter.

Electromagnetic fields (think cellphones) also have taken the rap, but to date, no conclusive scientific evidence supports the claim. Some rumors about things that cause cancer, such as tight underwired bras and antiperspirants, are just funny. These rumors have no basis in fact, much like the old myths that claimed illness was caused by the brisk night air or excessive personal hygiene.

Here's something else that doctors know for certain: Cancer is not contagious. You didn't "catch" it from anyone else, and your family and friends can't get it from you.

Finally, no one disputes that having cancer causes stress. The National Cancer Institute reports that that the stress can impact how well the body responds to infection and disease, including cancer, but to date no evidence exists that stress is directly responsible for causing cancer.

Research, of course, continues.

Types of cancer

Cancer is not just one single disease. It's actually many different diseases, each one complex in its own way. Here is a list of some of the different types of cancer. Keep in mind that each type of cancer also has subtypes.

- Bone cancers
- Brain tumors
- Breast cancers
- Endocrine system cancers
- Gastrointestinal cancers
- Gynecologic cancers
- Head and neck cancers
- Leukemia
- Lung cancers
- Lymphomas
- Myelomas (bone marrow cancers)
- Pediatric cancers
- Penile cancer
- Prostate cancer
- Sarcomas
- Skin cancers
- Testicular cancer
- Thyroid cancer
- Urinary tract cancers

Table 7-1 lists both the most common cancers afflicting men and women and the leading causes of cancer deaths in both populations.

Table 7-1	Three Most Common Cancers and Leading Cause of Cancer Deaths, by Gender (per 100,000 People)			
Men		**Women**	
Most Common Cancers	*Leading Causes of Cancer Death*	*Most Common Cancers*	*Leading Causes of Cancer Death*
Prostate (137.7)	Lung (62.0)	Breast (123.1)	Lung (38.6)
Lung (78.2)	Prostate (22.0)	Lung (54.1)	Breast (22.2)
Colorectal (49.2)	Colorectal (19.1)	Colorectal (37.1)	Colorectal (13.1)

Source: United States Cancer Statistics: 2009 Incidence and Mortality, U.S. Centers for Disease Control and Prevention

Differentiating among tumors

The types of cancer listed in the previous section are named for common sites where various cancers originate. Many of these cancers may spread, or metastasize — to other sites. For example, a breast cancer may spread to the lungs, bones, or brain.

When several organs are affected by cancer when you are diagnosed, a pathologist — a doctor who studies tissues with a microscope — establishes the site of the cancer's origin. If you are diagnosed with lung cancer that has metastasized to the adrenal glands, you won't hear the doctors say you have cancer of the adrenal glands. They will say you have lung cancer that has spread, because cancer is always defined according to the primary tumor. And if cancer comes back, it usually is not a new cancer; it contains the same cells found in the original tumor, even if the disease now is in a different part of the body.

When a cancer has spread, usually the outcome is not as favorable, and treatment may change as well. With few exceptions, the focus of treatment for metastasized cancer is more systemic, involving the whole body. Although important exceptions do exist, local treatments, such as surgery or radiation, generally are used for relief of symptoms.

Considering Risk Factors

Right now, doctors know that about 10 percent of all cancers are genetic, or inherited. But if only about 10 percent of cancers can be blamed on genetics, what factors contribute to cancer in the other 90 percent of the population?

There's no clear-cut answer, but this section discusses several well-known factors that may increase the risk of cancer.

Looking at genetic causes

As scientists begin to understand the human genome more thoroughly, they are slowly but steadily recognizing the genetic mutations that result in cancers. Research is under way right now to try to identify the precise locations of gene abnormalities that lead to cancers. When the locations are mapped, the goal will become to find ways to target these abnormalities with treatments that won't harm other organs.

The more predictable gene abnormalities that scientists detect, the more effective genetic screening becomes, so people at risk for cancer can be identified and treated before cancer develops. For example, mutations of two genes (known as BRCA-1 and BRCA-2) have been connected to the development of breast and ovarian cancer. There are families with strong histories of pancreatic cancer, malignant melanoma, colorectal, and other cancers. These families have mutations in other specific genes.

If you or your family members have a significant family history of any type of cancer, you want to speak with your doctor about genetic screening, which also can determine other known genetic abnormalities associated with inherited syndromes.

Looking at behavioral or environmental factors

People have long linked certain "undesirable" behaviors with getting ill. Although many of these connections are laughable (going outside with wet hair will make you sick, or cracking your knuckles will give you arthritis, for example), research has shown a relationship link between certain behaviors or environmental exposures and cancer.

Maybe you smoke, despite knowing that scientists have proven a correlation between smoking and lung cancer. Maybe you sunbathe without protection, despite knowing that doing so puts you at risk for skin cancers. If you develop cancer, does that mean you're to blame? No. Not everyone with a risk factor like smoking (or even with several risk factors) actually gets cancer. In fact, many people who have identified risk factors never develop cancer. Conversely, some people who have no known risk factors at all do develop cancer. The only explanation that makes sense is that some complex series of circumstances come into play at the cellular level that cause one person rather than another to develop cancer. In addition, certain risks that themselves are not true carcinogens track with the risk of cancer.

✔ **Using tobacco:** The National Cancer Institute reports that a third of all cancer deaths each year are due to using tobacco products — smoking or using smokeless tobacco — and being exposed to second-hand smoke. Though smokers are at the highest risk for lung cancer, they also are at higher risk for developing other kinds of cancer. The good news is that soon after a smoker quits, the risk of developing cancer begins to drop.

The first study reporting a connection between smoking and cancer was published in 1950. However, astute physicians practicing in the late 1700s noted an increase in polyps among snuff users (snuff was a powdered tobacco that users sniffed) and pipe smokers.

✔ **Eating an unhealthy diet, not getting enough exercise, and being overweight:** For years, researchers and laypeople alike have known that being overweight or obese, eating a high-fat, high-calorie diet, and not engaging in regular physical activity are bad for you, leading to conditions like heart disease, increasing your risk for high blood pressure and stroke, and making it more likely you'll develop diabetes. But they also increase your risk of certain kinds of cancers. The following cancers are associated with being overweight or obese; several are also associated with not getting enough physical activity:

- Breast cancer
- Colorectal cancer
- Endometrial cancer
- Esophageal cancer
- Kidney cancer
- Pancreatic cancer

The American Institute for Cancer Research reports that eating a diet high in vegetables, fruits, whole grains, and beans; maintaining a healthy weight; exercising regularly; and not smoking can lower cancer risk.

✔ **Drinking alcohol in excess:** The National Institute on Alcohol Abuse and Alcoholism estimates that 2 to 4 percent of all cancer cases are thought to be caused by excessive consumption of alcohol. What's "excessive"? That depends on many factors — gender, body weight, and family history among them. You probably know better than anyone else when your drinking is out of control.

✔ **Ultraviolet (UV) radiation:** The Skin Cancer Foundation has declared that skin cancer has reached epidemic proportions. In the past ten years, the number of cases of melanoma — the most serious form of skin cancer — has grown more than any other form of cancer. The Foundation's first rule of protection is this: Don't sunbathe.

✔ **Chemicals:** Today, most scientists agree that exposure to some pesticides, metals, and chemicals — such as polychlorinated biphenyls and other mixtures of toxic chemicals — may increase the risk of cancer. That also holds true for additives and for the natural chemicals found in some foods. (That said, some natural chemicals found in fruits and vegetables work in the body to fight cancer.)

✔ **X-ray procedures and medical radiation:** Radiation therapy treatments, which can damage healthy cells, also carry a slight risk — but, generally, the benefits of treatment are thought to outweigh the risks. If you are considering going through radiation therapy, your radiation oncologist can help you quantify what the risks of damage to healthy cells may be in your case.

✔ **Hormone replacement therapy (HRT):** For years, doctors routinely prescribed HRT for menopausal women. In 2002, The *Journal of the American Medical Association* published the results of a study on conjugated estrogens plus progestins (a type of hormone replacement therapy) that was halted by the National Institutes of Health after safety monitors realized that the participants receiving the drug had more incidents of breast cancer and other life-threatening diseases than those receiving the placebo. Still, some forms of short-term hormone replacement therapy may be helpful for some women suffering from extreme symptoms of menopause. If you are experiencing extreme symptoms, by all means speak with your doctor.

✔ **Having had cancer before:** People who survive cancer are at greater risk for the cancer coming back or for a second type of cancer developing. This increased risk is due both to the effects of cancer treatment as well as the factors (underlying genetics, unhealthy behaviors, exposure to carcinogens) that made them susceptible to cancer in the first place.

To improve chances for survival and to improve quality of life after a cancer diagnosis, eliminate unhealthy behaviors and replace them with healthy behaviors: If you smoke, quit. If you are overweight, adopt a lifestyle that supports healthy food choices and regular exercise. And, of course, follow up with your health care provider.

Controversy — sometimes the raging variety — has circled all around almost every risk factor listed here. One study shows this to be true, the next study shows that. When all is said and done regarding risk factors, it makes sense to want to improve your odds, to be aware of legitimate dangers to your health. Medical science has proven that changes in some personal behaviors can decrease the risk of cancer.

Fighting Back: Your Immune System and Treatment Options

Medical science is currently learning about and testing some ways to turn off the misguided cells that undergo a mutation and get busy transforming into cancer cells that attack the body. Today, chemotherapy and radiation are the time-tested standard treatments for most cancers. Many people diagnosed with cancer have both treatments, sometimes concurrently and sometimes one after the other. Some people have just one.

Basically, most chemotherapy is systemic; it involves any number of anticancer drugs that sweep through every cell in the body. In contrast, most radiation therapy is local or regional, meaning treatments are aimed specifically at the site of a tumor or at nearby places the tumor may have spread.

Your immune system

Marvel that it is, the body is programmed to fight infection and disease. Scientists think that the body fights cancer the same way it tries to protect you from viruses. How the immune system works is complicated. Here's an action-packed scenario of how your immune system works (see Figure 7-1):

1. **When a white blood cell known as a macrophage finds a virus, the macrophage devours and digests the virus.**

   The good guys don't always wear white hats, but your white blood cells are often heroes.

2. **Flaunting its victory, the macrophage displays bits of the virus on its surface.**

   These shreds of virus are known as *antigens*.

3. **A particular "helper" T cell notices the antigens on the surface of the macrophage and attaches itself.**

   A T cell is another type of white blood cell.

4. **Working together, the macrophage and the T cell produce several chemical substances that result in intercellular communication.**

5. **One of these substances sends signals to other helper T cells and also calls for help from "killer" T cells.**

   Both types of cells begin to multiply.

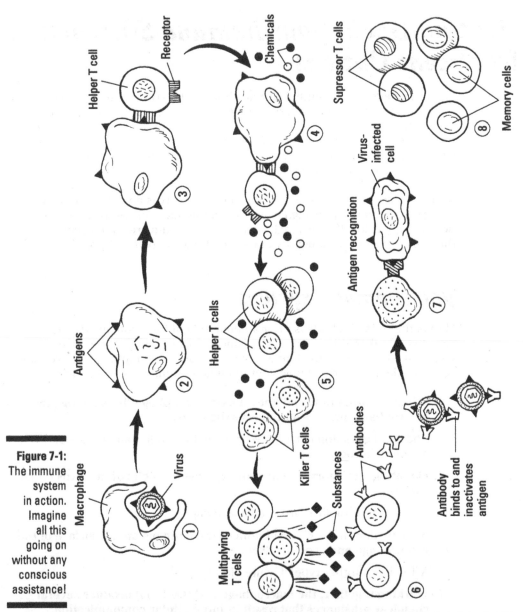

Figure 7-1:
The immune
system
in action.
Imagine
all this
going on
without any
conscious
assistance!

Illustration by Kathryn Born, MA

6. **The multiplying T cells release substances that cause additional helper cells to multiply and also to produce antibodies that bind to antigens.**

These antibodies enable the macrophages to destroy viruses more easily. They also signal blood components, called *complement*, to further damage the viruses.

7. The killer T cells scout around for additional cells in the area that have come under attack by viruses, and they repeat their good works.

8. When the immune system determines that the infection is under control, "suppressor" T cells move in and turn off the other cells.

Sentries, in the form of memory cells, stay on duty just in case the same virus mounts another attack.

Sounds something like an adventure movie, doesn't it?

Looking to the future: Ongoing research

Key weapons in the fight against cancer are research and the development of new treatments based on new discoveries. This section identifies two areas that are currently of particular interest to scientists.

Genetic culprits

Research continues into the genes and gene products that have been identified as causes of cancer in some people. For example, scientists know that two genes — *BRCA-1* and *BRCA-2* — are connected to the development of breast and ovarian cancers. Also, a gene known as *HER2/neu*, which helps regulate cell growth, may, if altered, cause particularly aggressive tumor cells. Genes that lead to the growth of blood vessels are also a research target, because blood vessels play a critical role in the *metastatic process* — the process by which cancer spreads from one organ to another.

Cancers caused by genes and gene products may not readily respond to standard chemotherapy treatments, but in some instances new drugs are available, and others are in development. For instance, in clinical trials the drug Herceptin (trastuzumab) has been shown to slow the growth of cancerous tumors in some women who test positive for abnormalities in the HER2/neu gene.

Many doctors believe that the future of oncology lies in identifying additional genetic changes that result in cancer and in developing new drugs aimed at those genes.

Developing fortified antibodies

Another important and growing focus of research aims at identifying tumor *antigens* that are characteristic of various malignant cells. After identifying these tumor antigens, the goal is to develop fortified antibodies to fight them. This follows the basic principle of treating an infection with antibiotics.

This targeted therapy would use multiple vectors armed with radioactive materials, antibiotics, or chemotherapy drugs to deliver a death blow to the cancer cells. A compound injected into the bloodstream would target a specific cancer cell type, wherever it may be in the body.

In principle, this type of therapy should work, but the catch is in identifying the antigen, fabricating an antibody, and uniting it with a radioactive material or chemo agent that won't damage any other cells in the body. The principle is simple, but the execution is complex.

As you may expect, the immune system goes after early cancer cells and destroys them whenever possible. Sometimes, that's not possible — for example, when overwhelming numbers of cancer cells exist or the cells have mutated in such a way that the immune system does not detect them, which allows the cells to evade immune surveillance.

In a situation where rapidly dividing cancer cells are at work in a body with an impaired immune system, the outlook can be grim. That said, doctors already have some weapons that help to boost an ailing immune system or enable the immune system to focus attention specifically on the cancerous cells. Eventually, they hope to develop even more weapons that will lend additional reinforcement to the troops already on duty.

Chemotherapy

Chemotherapy, or anticancer drug therapy, is a systemic treatment for cancer, which means that chemotherapy drugs move through the bloodstream to all parts of the body.

Time was when the word chemotherapy elicited almost as much fear as the word cancer. People heard "chemotherapy" and shuddered, because this particular treatment had a reputation for being as hard on the body as cancer itself. In some circles today, chemotherapy still is thought of as poison.

No doubt about it, chemotherapy is strong medicine. It has to be. The job of chemotherapy is to cure or control cancer, a disease that kills 1,500 Americans every day, according to the National Cancer Institute. One big reason more people don't die of cancer is the effectiveness of chemotherapy.

There's no question that undergoing chemotherapy can be rough. But many drugs have been developed to help offset some of the more disabling side effects of chemotherapy. Also, for a host of reasons, every individual responds to chemotherapy differently, so "rough" can range from profound fatigue to hospitalization. You may want to decide that instead of fearing chemotherapy, you will simply respect it for its power — and its possibilities.

Radiation

Radiation therapy is a local, or site-specific, treatment for cancer. Radiation may shrink or eradicate tumors, and it kills cancer cells that may linger after a tumor has been removed surgically.

Radiation has been used to treat cancer and other diseases for more than 100 years. Three discoveries, all of which occurred in the years just preceding 1900, led to radiation therapy: x-rays, radioactivity, and radium. In the early years of the 20th century, surgeons typically administered a single massive blast of radiation to a patient's body. Sometimes, miraculously, that worked — but often these earliest treatments were not successful.

That was then. Today, between 50 and 60 percent of all cancer patients undergo some form of radiation therapy. Science, as they say, marches on. Sophisticated machines deliver carefully calibrated doses of external beam radiation to a precise site anywhere in the body. Another form of radiation therapy, called *brachytherapy,* uses radioactive wires, seeds, or rods that are placed in the body close to the site of the tumor or directly into it.

Although the idea of radiation therapy can be scary, the reality is that this time-tested form of treatment is powerful and offers hope to people with cancer.

Linking the Mediterranean Diet to Cancer Prevention

Chemo and radiation therapy can cause changes in your eating habits, for a variety of reasons. In some cases, the treatment itself is responsible. In others, fatigue from the treatments can leave you too tired to eat, or the treatment itself can alter your taste for food. All of these possibilities are bad, because good nutrition is especially important during cancer treatments. Here are some reasons why:

✔ Eating well helps you keep your energy up.

✔ Good nutrition helps you manage side effects.

✔ A healthy diet can help your body fend off infection.

Whether you're undergoing treatment for cancer or want to reduce your risk for recurrence, good nutrition is key. The Mediterranean diet offers nutrient benefits for cancer prevention as well as improving your lifespan. The incidence of cancer in the Mediterranean is lower than in the UK and United States, and the specific cancers involved, like bowel, breast, and prostate, have been attributed to dietary causes.

Researchers out of Greece and Harvard who published work in the journal *Cancer Epidemiology, Biomarkers, and Prevention* estimate that up to 25 percent of incidences of colorectal cancer, 15 percent of breast cancer, and 10 percent of endometrial, prostate, and pancreatic cancer could be prevented with adherence to a Mediterranean diet. Let food be your medicine (in addition, of course, to whatever treatment your primary physician recommends)!

Here are some things you can do:

- **Eat less meat.** If you do, research shows your risk for cancer is reduced, up to 50 percent according to some studies. Instead of eating meat, get your protein from fish, eggs, nuts, seeds, and grains, all of which contain protein. Mediterranean favorites include fish like salmon, tuna, sardines; nuts like walnuts or pistachios; and grains like bulgur and quinoa.

- **Eat more fruits and veggies.** Flavonoids found in many plant-based foods are antioxidants and contain additional compounds that may prevent the risk of cells turning cancerous. Fiber found in fruits, veggies, and legumes can also help reduce the risk of certain types of cancers. Refer to Chapters 9 through 11 for more on the common plant-based foods in the Mediterranean diet. Remember, the more variety, the better for your health because you also obtain a variety of nutrition.

- **More olive oil, please!** Olive oil is a healthy monounsaturated fat that helps fight inflammation and risk for developing cancer, especially when combined with a diet that avoids high-fat meat, dairy, and butter. Chapter 8 delves more into olive oil, how to include it in your diet, and how much is enough for your diet and your health.

Part III

Digging Deeper into the Mediterranean Diet

Five Foods High on the Must-Eat List

✔ **Olive oil:** If one food stands out in the Mediterranean diet, it's olive oil, which gets credit for a number of health benefits, like reducing cholesterol, protecting against the build up of plaque in your arteries, reducing the risk of cancer, lowering blood pressure, improving brain function and reducing the risk of Alzheimer's, improving blood glucose control, fighting osteoporosis, and more.

✔ **Walnuts:** Walnuts' antioxidant content is almost double that of all other nuts, and they contain mostly healthy fats, the kind that reduce inflammation, reduce the risk of heart disease and certain types of cancer, benefit brain health, and offer protection from cognitive decline.

✔ **Legumes:** They're a great source of protein and fiber; can be a substitute for higher-fat proteins and refined grains; and are inexpensive and readily available. They also lower bad cholesterol, help control blood glucose levels, reduce risk for heart disease and cancer, and have a boatload of antioxidants, vitamins, and minerals.

✔ **Seafood:** In addition to being a lean protein, seafood's main benefit is its omega-3 fatty acid content, which helps reduce inflammation throughout the body, lowers the risk of depression, improves visual and neurological development of infants in utero, possibly lowers triglycerides and the risk for heart disease, and reduces the risk of Alzheimer's disease.

✔ **Wine:** Okay, so wine isn't a must-eat, but the fact that it's important enough to warrant placement on the Mediterranean diet food pyramid speaks both to its health benefits and its role as a reminder that the Mediterranean diet isn't about deprivation but enjoying all the good things that life has to offer.

Find a complete list of key foods on the Mediterranean and the nutrients they offer at www.dummies.com/extras/mediterraneandiet.

In this part . . .

✔ Discover the different varieties of olive oil, the health benefits it offers, how much a healthy diet should include, and how to use it in cooking.

✔ Distinguish the difference between nuts, seeds, and legumes; identify the nutrients found in the varieties featured in the Mediterranean diet; and learn how to incorporate them into your cooking.

✔ Find out why fruits and vegetables play such an important role in health eating, what the key nutrients in the varieties prominently featured in the Mediterranean diet are, and how to get the required seven to ten servings in each day.

✔ Include whole grains, including all the benefits they offer, into your diet.

✔ Dive into lean protein sources, especially the Mediterranean favorites — fish and seafood — but also poultry and lean meats, as you rethink portion sizes for a healthier meal.

✔ Find out why drinking a glass of red wine with your meal can improve both your mood and your health.

Chapter 8

The Miracle of Olive Oil

. . . .

In This Chapter

▶ Identifying key components and varieties of olive oil

▶ Recognizing why olive oil is an important part of the Mediterranean diet

▶ Discovering how to use olive oil in your diet and cooking, without going overboard

. . . .

Olive oil is the secret sauce of the Mediterranean diet. Although Western diets feature hydrogenated oils and saturated fats from animal sources, olive oil — the staple of Mediterranean cuisine — is rich in plant-based mono-unsaturated fatty acids that are chockfull of heart health benefits. Making the swap can improve your health without compromising on flavor that other fat sources add to your meals.

Similar to all the nutritious components of the Mediterranean diet, olive oil is widely used because it's locally procured and processed. Instead of relying on commercially prepared foods that need to travel long distances, the people in the Mediterranean rely on their natural surroundings to provide many of the staples of their diet, like locally grown fruits and vegetables, olive oil processed from olive trees in their backyard, and fish caught nearby. This focus on local is why much of the Mediterranean cuisine is comprised of foods that are identical or close to how they are found in nature and provide the best nutrition nature can offer! This chapter introduces you to the components and different varieties of olive oil and explains how to best use it without overdoing it.

You may be thinking, "Okay, this sounds great and all, but doesn't oil add a lot of calories to my diet?" Yes, oil is a calorie-dense food. For your weight and health, it's important to keep calories, from whatever you eat, in check. But too little fat isn't healthy for you, either, and getting enough from the right sources can help you maintain your weight and reduce your risk for disease.

Taking a Deeper Look at Olive Oil

There's much more to olive oil than simply picking up any random bottle at your grocery store to use on your salad. Of course, if you did that instead of using a bottled ranch or buttermilk dressing, you'd probably have a leg up when it comes to your health. But if you want to know more, you're in the right place. This section provides insight into the varieties you can choose, gives you a rundown of the healthy fat found in olive oil, and explains why olive oil is beneficial for your heart and body. You also discover what olive oil *is not* and how the thing that distinguishes it from typical fats of a Western diet makes it the healthy choice to add to any dish on your menu.

Discovering what's in olive oil

All oils, including olive oil, contain three types of fat: monounsaturated, poly-unsaturated, and saturated fat.

What makes one oil better for you than another is the proportion of these types of fat within the oil. Olive oil is considered mainly a monounsaturated fat because 1 tablespoon contains about 120 calories and 14 grams of fat, broken down in the following way (for extra virgin olive oil):

- **10 grams of monounsaturated fat:** About 55 to 85 percent of olive oil is comprised of the monounsaturated fat *oleic acid*. Monounsaturated fats, or MUFAs, are particularly beneficial for your cholesterol levels.

- **2 grams of polyunsaturated fat:** Polyunsaturated fat includes *alpha-lin-oleic acid*, an omega-3 fatty acid, and *linoleic acid*, an omega-6 fatty acid. These types of fats are generally a plus for your cholesterol levels and heart health, too.

- **2 grams of saturated fat:** You may be surprised that olive oil also con-tains saturated fat, the type of solid fat associated with higher choles-terol levels. But the proportion is small, and research suggests saturated fat from vegetable sources doesn't have the same harmful impact on heart health as that from animal sources (like butter, lard, other dairy, and meat products).

The calories in olive oil all come from fat, meaning olive oil naturally doesn't contain any other macronutrients, like carbohydrates or protein, nor does it contain any cholesterol or sodium. However, it is a source of the following:

- **Vitamin E (10 percent RDA per tablespoon):** Vitamin E is a fat-soluble antioxidant that may help prevent heart disease, certain types of can-cers, and skin conditions, as well as enhance immune function.

✔ **Vitamin K (7 percent RDA per tablespoon):** A fat-soluble vitamin necessary for calcium absorption and bone health, vitamin K is also responsible for blood clotting and promotes blood vessel health.

✔ **Polyphenols (plant-based compounds like *tyrosol* and *hydroytryosol*):** Antioxidants play a role in reducing inflammation, reducing your risk for cancer and heart disease, and lowering blood pressure and cholesterol.

✔ **Carotenoids (beta-carotene, lutein, and zeaxanthin):** The fat-soluble pigment that's responsible for olive oil's yellow-orange color, these antioxidants promote eye health and protect the lining of your arteries from oxidation, improving heart health. Vitamin A also boosts your immune function in general.

✔ **Chlorophyll:** A pigment in olive oil responsible for the greenish color which may or may not have antioxidant benefits (it's unclear!)

I delve more into the health benefits of olive oil later in this section.

When you consider using any type of oil or butter, remember that they are all a combination of various types of fat. For your reference, Table 8-1 offers a breakdown of common items and shows how other oils and fat sources match up.

Table 8-1	Fat Source Breakdown			
Source	*Saturated*	*Monounsaturated*	*Polyunsaturated*	*Trans*
Olive oil	2	10	2	0
Canola oil	1	9	4	0
Safflower oil	1	10	2	0
Margarine (Stick)	4	4	3	3
Butter	7.5	3	0.5	0

Source: Based on USDA Nutrient Database values

Drizzling down the varieties

All olive oil is not created equal. Many factors impact the taste, color, and aroma, and these factors result in hundreds of varieties of olive oil. You can compare the varieties of olive oil to the many types of wine that are produced, each being impacted by type of grape, growing conditions, harvest time, and so on.

From tree to bottle

Before drizzling down the varieties of olive oil, you may be curious to know how it's made, from tree to bottle. Keep reading:

1. **Mediterranean olive trees start bearing fruit, olives, after about five years.**

   Olive trees have a very impressive lifespan. Some trees live and produce for several hundred years! The olive is a green *drupe* (fruit surrounding a single pit), and as it ripens, it turns black or deep purple.

2. **Olives are harvested, using a tree-shaking device or by being hand-picked (labels often differentiate between the two), and the stems, leaves, and twigs are removed.**

   Olives contain the highest concentration of polyphenols, or antioxidants, for about two to three weeks as they ripen. Ideally they're harvested during that time. The more ripe, the more oil an olive contains as well, but the best oil comes from olives that are a reddish color (not fully ripened).

3. **Rollers crush the olives into a paste, which is then cold pressed and sent through a centrifuge device to separate the oil out.**

   The solid matter that remains is known as *pomace* and is often pressed again for oil that is classified as *olive-pomace oil*. For the most part, olive-pomace oil is used commercially, meaning that you won't see it on your grocery store shelf.

4. **The oil is refined in various ways to reduce acidity and to remove pesticides.**

   This process also removes chlorophyll and nutrients.

5. **The processed oil is stored at about 65 degrees Fahrenheit before being bottled and shipped to market.**

Unlike wine, olive oil labels won't always list the type of olive used. Nor does olive oil get better with age! In fact, the older it gets, the more the polyphenol content and health benefits decrease. Experts suggest a bottle of olive oil has a two-year shelf life, maximum. For the most part, consume olive oil within 12 to 18 months after harvest. Because you may not be privy to this info, go by the expiration date on the bottle.

The varieties of olive oil are due to the following:

- Type of olive
- Growing conditions of the olive tree (that is, location, soil, environmental, and weather)
- How the olives are harvested (that is, the ripeness of the olive, and the time between harvest and pressing)
- The method by which olives are pressed, stored, and packaged for sale

Most of the world's olive oil is produced in Spain, Italy, and Greece. Oils from different countries or areas can be blended together. Specific regional varieties, or estate olive oils using olives that are hand-pressed from a single farm, are also available. As you go from former to latter in that list, the uniqueness goes up, and so does the price tag!

The International Olive Oil Council (IOOC) sets standards that most countries use to grade olive oils. The U.S. Department of Agriculture uses its own standards, but these are similar to the IOOC standards. In the following sections, I define the grades of olive oil and what you can expect with each.

Grades mainly have to do with the level of processing the olives undergo to become oil. At the head of the class, the extra virgin and virgin olive oils are the result of one cold press of olives, and no further refining — with chemicals or heat — occurs afterwards, helping the oil to maintain its nutritional value and flavor. When refined further, oils lose their "virginity." The grades are also defined by their acidity; the lower acidity, the better the taste!

Nutritionally speaking, not much of a difference in fat content exists among the oils except those that are more heavily refined contain less polyphenols. The more polyphenols, the better for your health. But you're not solely choosing olive oil for the antioxidants (and many other foods on the Mediterranean diet plan contain a higher percentage of polyphenols). You're choosing it to replace more saturated, less heart-healthy sources of fat like butter in your diet.

Extra virgin

Extra virgin is the finest of the oils and has the least acidity (no more than 0.8 percent acidity). Premium extra virgin olive oil has even lower acidity. The extra virgins can be a pale yellow to bright green color. The deeper the golden color, the more intense the fruity flavor. Extra virgin olive oil is also more likely to have a high concentration of polyphenols.

Use this type of oil straight up! Because of its superior flavor and aroma, use it as a dip for bread, over salads, or as a condiment in uncooked dishes. Doing so lets you appreciate what it has to offer.

When purchasing extra virgin olive oil, choose a bottle with dark glass and store it in a cool, dry place. Doing so helps prevent oxidation of the oil (which alters its chemical composition) and optimizes its shelf-life. If you don't use the oil often, buy smaller bottles, because the more the oil is exposed to air, the more the flavor decreases.

Fino (fine) oils

Fine virgin oil is usually a combination of extra virgin and virgin olive oils. The acidity level can't exceed 1.5 percent, according to the IOOC standards. You use these just as you would extra virgin.

Virgin

The virgin oils have acidity levels between 1 and 3 percent. Although they have enough flavor to be enjoyed uncooked, they are typically used in cooking.

Light oil

The "light" designation doesn't refer to the oil's fat content; it refers to its lighter color and flavoring. Light olive oil has the same amount of calories and fat as any of the oils, but it's undergone filtration after the first press to remove most of the flavor and coloring (without heat or chemical processes).

This filtration makes light oil a good choice to use for baking and cooking when the olive oil flavoring isn't desirable. It's also a good oil to use when you need to cook at a high heat because the processing gives the oil a higher smoke point. Both virgin and non-virgin oils can hold this classification.

Refined oils

When heat and chemical processes come into play to refine oils further, they lose the title *virgin*. This extra processing can happen if virgin oils have too high an acidity, poor flavor, or poor aroma.

Processing into refined oils renders them flavorless, odorless, and colorless, which gives them a longer shelf-life. They're often used in combination with virgin olive oils when cooking or in items that are labeled "packed in oil."

Organic olive oils

Organic olive oil ensures the product is free of chemicals. A product labeled as organic ensures that only natural methods were used during growth and harvest of the olives. However, getting an organic certification is expensive, and these oils can cost you up to 75 percent more per bottle than a conventional oil.

Conventional olive oil, especially ones that are extra virgin, may be just as pure as the "organic" brands.

Understanding the benefits of olive oil

The benefits you get from using olive oil go beyond the nutrients it adds; you also need to take into account the not-so-good stuff that you reduce or eliminate when you use this fat source in place of others! Olive oil, on its own and in combination with additional nutritious dietary changes, has been researched extensively and found to have an abundance of health benefits:

✔ **Reduces cholesterol.** The MUFAs, which comprise 75 percent of olive oil, lower your "bad" (LDL) cholesterol and raise your "good" (HDL) cholesterol, which has a heart-protective impact. To have this effect, use olive oil as a replacement for saturated fats and hydrogenated oils in your diet.

✔ **Protects against oxidative stress.** In the European Union, olive oil is qualified to hold this claim: "Olive oil polyphenols contribute to the protection of blood lipids from oxidative stress." Oxidation is the process by which plaque builds up in your arteries, increasing your risk for heart attack, stroke, and death from cardiovascular disease. Both polyphenols and vitamin E can help prevent LDL cholesterol oxidation.

✔ **Reduces risk of cancer.** Researchers out of the University of Athens conducted a review of studies and concluded that higher olive oil intake was associated with a reduced risk for cancer. One compelling study, conducted at Northwestern University Feinberg School of Medicine, may have found the mechanism for this in breast cancer specifically. Oleic acid seems to block a protein that boosts growth of breast cancer cells.

✔ **Lowers blood pressure.** Multiple large-scale studies, including the European Prospective Investigation into Cancer and Nutrition (EPIC) study, have found an inverse relationship between olive oil and blood pressure (that is, as olive oil consumption goes up, blood pressure goes down). This relationship is likely due to the action of both oleic acid and polyphenols in olive oil preventing oxidation of cholesterol, which leads to atherosclerosis and increased blood pressure.

✔ **Improves cognitive function.** Research shows that the type of fat you consume impacts your cognition and memory. A study tracking vascular risk factors published in *Neurology,* the medical journal for the American Academy of Neurology, found that olive oil has a specific impact. Those who had 2 to 3 tablespoons per day had lower chances for cognitive issues. In addition, a compound in olive oil called *oleocanthal* may protect nerve cells from damage due to Alzheimer's disease, improving outcomes.

✔ **Improves blood glucose control.** Current studies suggest that olive oil can help diabetes risk factors. It's not a direct causation, but the effect of having a calorie-controlled, good-tasting, heart-healthy, fat-rich diet versus a low-fat diet resulted in better blood glucose control according to a study published in the journal for the German Diabetes Association.

✔ **Fights osteoporosis.** People who consume a Mediterranean diet enriched with olive oil may have better bone health, according to at least one study published in the *Journal of Clinical Endocrinology and Metabolism.* The participants' levels of calcium and serum *osteocalcin,* a protein important to bone creation, were higher than the levels in the control group.

The power of smell

When dissecting olive oil's components and what it can replace in your diet, olive oil is clearly a nutritious choice. But could the oil's aroma unlock a key to its weight-loss potential as well? Research out of the German Research Center for Food Chemistry found that yes, olive oil can increase a person's feelings of satiety after a meal. Just by adding the aroma to a dish, participants consumed fewer calories, and their blood glucose response improved. Fluctuations in blood glucose are associated with cravings, and olive oil's aroma helped keep those in check as well.

The researchers realized they needed to take the study a step further. They also compared the response with canola oil, butter, and lard to see whether this effect was specific to olive oil. The study group that received the olive oil foods actually had greater increases in serotonin, a hormone that helps you feel full, compared to groups receiving foods with the other fats. When the participants felt satisfied, they were more likely to reduce their calorie intake the rest of the day and more likely to lose weight.

Although the sample size was small, this study is just another example that hunger and fullness is driven by more than the components of food. There is also a clear psychological factor as well. And maybe even the aroma compound in olive oil, *hexanal,* which smells like freshly cut grass, can also help you in the weight-loss department.

✔ **Reduces inflammation.** The compound oleocanthal prevents the pro-inflammatory activity of an enzyme. It acts as a naturally occurring ibuprofen to help reduce symptoms of arthritis.

✔ **Acts as an antibacterial.** Olive oil polyphenols may inhibit the growth of bacteria *H. pylori,* which causes stomach ulcers and promotes stomach cancer.

✔ **Enhances digestion and absorption of nutrients.** The fat-soluble vitamins A, D, E, and K, some of which are present in olive oil, require fat in order to be absorbed. Olive oil helps facilitate digestion and absorption of these essential nutrients.

If you treat olive oil as an addition to your current diet without making other changes, you'll probably get more calories, fat, and less healthy benefits than you bargained for. The goal is to use olive oil as part of a diet rich in fruits, vegetables, and legumes, and low in fatty meats and dairy — which describes the Mediterranean diet perfectly!

Olive Oil and the Mediterranean Diet

The Dietary Guidelines for Americans suggest that, on average, about 30 percent of your calories should come from fat. With the Mediterranean diet, you get up to 40 percent of your calories from fat. It may seem like a paradox that a diet richer in fat is healthier for you. But it's time to dispel the old nutrition myth that fat is bad! Of course, where the fat comes from is a key factor. Mostly all of the fat calories from the Mediterranean diet come from olive oil, fish oil, and nuts.

Actually, in the 1960s, about 45 percent of Americans' calories came from fats and oils — a time when the obesity rate was below 15 percent. Today, when closer to 30 percent of calories come from fat, about one-third of American adults are obese. What gives?

When people reduced fat intake, they did so across the board, cutting out sources of heart-healthy fats as well as unhealthy fats. This change occurred around the same time that we turned to consuming more refined carbohydrates, like white breads and other whole grains stripped of their nutrients, and sugary drinks, which are naturally low in fat. In addition, low-fat food products added refined carbohydrates back in for flavor. Compounding the problem was the fact that low-fat products are neither psychologically nor physically satisfying, making us prone to consuming larger portions to feel satisfied.

The shift away from all-natural foods that contain real ingredients instead of processed food is exactly what the Mediterranean diet is *not*. Nor does the Mediterranean diet isolate one food group as "good" or "bad," a tendency of traditional Western diets that hasn't helped our health or weight in the long haul.

The results of a large-scale study published in the *New England Journal of Medicine* in 2013 were so dramatic and foretelling that the researchers ended the study early to spread the word. This study followed about 7,500 people in Spain over the course of about five years. At the beginning of the study, the participants did not have heart disease. They were divided into three categories:

✔ **Category 1:** Mediterranean diet plus at least 4 tablespoons extra virgin olive oil every day

✔ **Category 2:** Mediterranean diet plus at least 30 grams of nuts every day

✔ **Category 3:** Low-fat diet

Those participants in the first two categories had a 25 to 30 percent lower risk of suffering heart attack and stroke. Few studies before this have established a direct link between diet and life-threatening occurrences. Typically, studies measure markers like cholesterol levels and weight, but experts close to the study suggest that diet can be a primary prevention against cardiac events like stroke. For more information on this study and other studies related to the Mediterranean diet or the foods on it, head to Chapter 18.

Consumption 101: How Much Is Too Much?

As with anything, eating too much olive oil isn't good for you. Although you need a certain amount of fat in your diet, getting too much contributes excess calories. And when you're eating more calories than your body needs or can use for energy, those calories can get stored as fat.

Fat is the most calorie-dense *macronutrient* (the three nutrients your body requires in the largest quantity) at 9 calories per gram. Protein and carbohydrates, on the other hand, have 4 calories per gram.

On the Mediterranean diet, about 30 to 40 percent of your calories come from fat, including olive oil and sources like fatty fish, nuts, seeds, and avocado, to name a few. Therefore, depending on the amount of calories you need, you can allot for different amounts. Table 8-2 gives you an example of how many fat grams you should eat daily, based on the total number of calories you consume per day. The amount of fat grams from olive oil equates to about half of your fat needs.

Table 8-2	How Much Olive Oil Should You Eat?	
Calories Per Day	*Total Grams of Fat Per Day*	*Suggested Olive Oil and Fat Grams*
1,500	58	2 tablespoons = 28 grams
1,800	70	2–3 tablespoons = 35 grams
2,100	82	3 tablespoons = 42 grams
2,400	93	3–4 tablespoons = 49 grams

When pouring directly into a dish or dipping bread, you may be soaking up more olive oil than you bargained for. Always measure out your portion ahead of time or use an olive oil mister (many brands are available in stores and online) to add a spray of flavor without worrying about adding too many calories or fat.

Cooking and Baking with Oils

Drizzling olive oil over salads and using it as a dip for breads are not the only easy ways to incorporate olive oil into your diet. Adding olive oil helps enhance the flavors and spices within any dish, adds body, and helps you feel more satisfied with what you're eating in general. You can use olive oil in a variety of ways when cooking or baking.

An oil's smoke point is the temperature at which the oil starts to smoke and break down into harmful substances (carcinogenic free radicals) as well as lose flavor. If you reach that point, discard the oil and whatever you've prepared in it. For olive oil, the smoke point is within a range about 375 to 410 degrees Fahrenheit, depending on the quality of oil. Virgin olive oils have a lower smoke point than others, so if you are cooking at high heats, consider using a fine virgin, a more refined olive oil, or canola oil, which has a higher smoke point.

Virgin olive oils also tend to lose their flavor more when heated, so they are best used in uncooked or low-heat dishes, drizzled on salads, and used for dips.

If you're replacing butter with olive oil, you need to use about only three-fourths the amount the recipe calls for. For example, if the recipe calls for 2 tablespoons butter, use 1½ tablespoons olive oil; if it requires 1 cup of butter, use ¾ cup olive oil, and so on.

The various ways you can use olive oil when cooking or baking are endless! Here are some suggestions (refer to Chapter 16 for specific ideas for different dishes):

- Use olive oil in a stir-fry dish with vegetables and seasonings.

- Brush fish or poultry with olive oil before grilling, or roast your fish or poultry in an olive oil–coated skillet.

- Spray a mist of olive oil over potatoes before baking, or whip it into mashed potatoes instead of butter.

- Drizzle olive oil onto whole wheat bread and toast to make croutons or sandwich bread.

- Use olive oil instead of butter in marinades, sauces, stocks, and stews.

- Make your own salad dressing or dips by combining extra virgin olive oil with other ingredients like vinegar, mustard, low-fat yogurt, mashed beans, herbs, and spices.

- Use light-flavored olive oil instead of butter for pancake and waffle batter and baking recipes like muffins, breads, and cakes.

Making infused olive oil

Herb or spice-infused olive oils typically carry a hefty price tag. Why not make your own at home to add a more robust flavor to your meals? Choose whatever fresh or dried herbs and spices you like — basil and garlic, for example, or rosemary and red pepper — and then follow these steps:

1. **Wash the fresh herbs and pat them dry. Combine them with your spices and/or dried herbs.**

2. **Warm the oil in a saucepan over low heat until warm.**

3. **Place the herbs and spices into a decorative bottle. Pour the warm oil over them and cover the bottle with a tight lid.**

4. **Place the bottle in a cool, dark place for a week.**

    Note: If you are using garlic, store the infused oil in the refrigerator to prevent food-borne illness.

5. **Strain the oil, removing and discarding the herbs and spices.**

Use the olive oil within one week. If you notice the oil begins to change color, discard it immediately.

Chapter 9

Nuts, Seeds, and Legumes

In This Chapter

▶ Getting back to nutrition basics with nuts, seeds, and legumes

▶ Understanding the most Mediterranean-friendly types and combos

▶ Discovering how to easily incorporate seeds, nuts, and legumes into your diet

Don't be fooled by the small size of nuts, seeds, and legumes: These three food groups are super strong when it comes to their nutrition power! Because the Mediterranean diet is mostly plant-based, you may think you'd be lacking in nutrients like protein, feeling sluggish, and constantly hungry. But nuts, seeds, and legumes know how to be the star in Mediterranean dishes, and when they're not the featured item on the place, they round out any meal with additional heart-healthy fats, protein, fiber, antioxidants, and plenty of vitamins and minerals. As you start decreasing the amount of meat and dairy you eat, supplementing with these versatile vegetarian foods helps boost your energy levels, keeps you satisfied, and adds unique flavors to your dishes.

This chapter breaks down the nuts, seeds, and legumes that are the MVPs of the Mediterranean diet and tells you how to start adding them to your meals today. If you've never explored the ways you can enjoy these foods, you are in for a treat!

Of course, no one got healthy by eating an excessive amount of any one food group. On that note, you'll also discover how to integrate nuts, seeds, and legumes in your diet in appropriate quantities and how you can best balance these foods with the other items on your plate. Finally, to maximize their nutrient benefit, you've got to know how to best choose and store these nuts, seeds, and legumes. This chapter covers that info, too.

Getting the Basics on Nuts, Legumes, and Seeds

Nuts, legumes, and seeds have been touted as "super foods" since way before the Mediterranean diet entered the spotlight. Before getting into the specific varieties common to the people who live around the Mediterranean sea, this section explains what these food groups are and identifies the health benefits that lie within. With this information in hand, you'll understand why these groups should be staples in your diet, too, instead of being relegated to a part of a snack you have from time to time.

Understanding what they are

Nuts and seeds and legumes can be very confusing to define because all nuts include a seed, but not all seeds are nuts. You think of almonds and pistachios as nuts, but they're really seeds from *drupes,* another category of fruit altogether (one in which the fruit surrounds a single pit). And you think a peanut is a nut, too, right? Think again — it's a legume.

What?! Take a breath and try not to get all caught up in the details. For education purposes, here are the true definitions of nuts, seeds, and legumes from a botanical sense (you'll notice some overlap between these, too):

- ✔ True *nuts* have a hard shell containing both the fruit and seed of a plant. The fruit does not open up to release the seed. Examples of true nuts include hazelnuts (one that's popular in the Mediterranean), chestnuts, hickory nuts, and acorns.

- ✔ *Seeds* refer to small plants containing embryos that are used to reproduce plants, fruits, and drupes. The seeds also contain a store of nutrients used by the plant to grow and develop. The nutrients within vary from species to species but are in the form of starches, oils, and proteins.

- ✔ *Legumes* are plants in the family *Fabaceae* and include the fruit or seeds or other edible part of that plant family. Legumes can be immature, like peas and green beans, which are harvested before maturation and are typically thought of as vegetables. When legumes are harvested after they've matured, they're dried seeds within pods, like beans, lentils, and peanuts, for example.

As I note earlier, the preceding are the botanical definitions. But each is referred to a bit differently from a culinary standpoint, which is the definition you're probably familiar with (which means you can go back to thinking of a peanut as a nut instead of a legume). From this point forward, I refer to them by their more familiar culinary uses. After all, that's why you're reading: to learn to incorporate these foods into your diet.

Tree nuts are one of the biggest allergens in America and refer to both true nuts and seeds, such as hazelnuts, almonds, Brazil nuts, cashews, pistachios, cashews, pecans, macadamias, and walnuts. The proteins in peanuts are very similar to those in tree nuts, which is why peanuts on their own are also in the top eight allergen list. If you are allergic to most nuts and seeds, don't worry! You can still get the nutrients within from other components of the Mediterranean diet, like olive oil, fatty fish, whole grains, and fruits and veggies.

Looking at their benefits

When you begin to look at the benefits offered by seeds, nuts, and legumes, you'll find that these small packages contain boatloads of nutrition. Depending on the variety, you get different benefits.

Following is a list of the nutrients found in seeds, nuts, and legumes, as well as their role in lowering your risk for heart disease, diabetes, and obesity:

- ✔ **Unsaturated fats:** Nuts and seeds contain both monounsaturated and polyunsaturated fats, which can help lower "bad" (LDL) cholesterol and improve heart health. The fat in nuts, when consumed with meals, also helps slow the absorption of blood sugar and, therefore, reduces spikes in blood glucose and cravings.

- ✔ **Omega-3 fatty acids:** Some nuts and seeds contain the best plant source of omega-3 fatty acids that money can buy (omega-3s are also found in many types of fish). In plants, the omega-3s appear primarily in the form of *alpha-linolenic acid* (ALA), which is integral for hormones that perform many functions like fighting inflammation; it can also help reduce your risk for heart disease and cancer.

- ✔ **Plant sterols and stanols:** These substances, found in nuts, seeds, and legumes, help prevent cholesterol from being absorbed into your blood stream. They're often added to margarines and orange juice, but they're naturally found in plant sources.

- ✔ **Fiber:** Fiber is the indigestible part of a carbohydrate that helps keep your cholesterol in check and helps regulate blood glucose. A study published in the *Journal of Nutrition* in 2012 found that adding just a half cup of cooked beans (rich in soluble fiber) per day reduced cholesterol levels by up to 8 percent over the course of 12 weeks. Fiber, no matter the kind, also helps keep you fuller longer, which may also help with weight control.

Here's another reason to go nuts: Research published in the *American Journal for Clinical Nutrition* found that adding an ounce of nuts to your daily intake as a substitute for fats found in meat or dairy was correlated with a lower risk of obesity and weight gain. The FDA has sanctioned this health claim on packages: "Scientific evidence suggests but does not prove that eating 1.5 ounces per day of most nuts, as part of a diet low in saturated fat and cholesterol, may reduce the risk of heart disease."

✔ **L-arginine:** *L-arginine* is an amino acid (a building block of protein) found naturally in nuts, seeds, and legumes. Your body uses it to make *nitric oxide,* a vasodilator (that is, it dilates blood vessels), which promotes healthy blood vessels and may help reduce blood pressure and risk for heart disease. L-arginine also functions in muscle building and repair.

L-arginine is used on its own and in combination with over-the-counter and prescription meds for a variety of reasons, from weight lifting to fighting infections. But it can be dangerous when taken in supplement form, so make sure to check with your doctor before doing so. But the natural kind found in nuts, seeds, and legumes is a-okay!

✔ **Protein:** Legumes — especially soy, but beans, too — are the greatest source of vegan protein. Nuts and seeds also contain smaller amounts of protein. Getting your fill can help you feel more satisfied longer and provide more energy, which can get you through your day. Legumes like beans are low in fat, offering a lean source of protein that makes sense at any meal.

✔ **Antioxidants, vitamins, and minerals:** Containing phytoestrogens like *lignans* (the component that makes plant walls rigid), vitamin E, folic acid, potassium, iron, and calcium, nuts, seeds, and legumes really do have it all! For more on what's found in each of the popular Mediterranean varieties of nuts and seeds and why these nutrients are good for your health, head to the next section.

Who says eating healthy needs to cost a lot of money? Nuts, seeds, and legumes are inexpensive, portable sources of good nutrition. So not only are they chockfull of nutrients that benefit your health, but they're also easy to take to work and school, in long car rides, and on the hiking trail. Because they are nonperishable and don't need to be refrigerated, nuts, seeds, and legumes make great snacks that can take you anywhere!

Cracking Down on the Nut and Seed Varieties

No matter what types of nuts and seeds you choose, you're doing yourself a favor and reaping loads of benefits, as the preceding section outlines. Also the more types you eat, the better variety of nutrients you get. But certain nuts and seeds fall in to the MVP — or Most Valuable Plants, Nuts & Seeds Class — category! In this section, I list the nuts and seeds that are essential to the Mediterranean diet, explain how they're commonly used in dishes, and tell you about specific bonuses they offer in the health and nutrition department.

Almonds

Although California is the number one producer of almonds in the world, these nuts are deep rooted in Mediterranean history and industries dating back thousands of years. Explorers ate this nut as they traveled between Asia and the Mediterranean on the Silk Road. And shortly afterward, almond trees were planted and flourished in Spain, Italy, Greece, and Morocco. The domesticated varieties have a sweet flavor, although the bitter varieties are also used in cooking.

Enjoying the health benefits

Almonds have been heavily researched for their health benefits, specifically in studies that investigate their ability to lower cholesterol and promote weight loss relative to lower-in-fat diets. Here are some highlights:

✔ Some theories suggest that the unique taste and texture of almonds may contribute to increased satiation and reduced calorie intake later on.

✔ Research suggests that the cell walls of almonds may prevent fat absorption. If this theory is true, almonds not only keep you satisfied, but they also provide less calories than other nuts or foods with the same amount of fat.

✔ Besides being a good source of nutrients typical to most nuts, almonds are a great source of vitamin E (a powerful antioxidant) and potassium (helps regulate blood pressure). These nutrients, combined with the almond's monounsaturated fat, help lower LDL cholesterol and reduce risk of atherosclerosis and heart disease. Vitamin E also can help boost immunity and prevent the signs of aging because of its role in cell regeneration.

✔ Almonds are a rich source of calcium for bone and heart health. In addition, almond milk can be consumed instead of dairy. See the next section for details.

Incorporating almonds into your diet

Although almonds are typically consumed in their raw form, they are extremely versatile and frequently used in cooking. Here's are some ideas for how you can incorporate them into your diet:

✔ Almonds are great to eat raw, roasted, in slices or slivers, and even come cocoa dusted! Add these to oatmeal, salad, yogurt, rice pilaf, and chicken and fish dishes, You can also eat them on their own as a snack.

You can also use chopped almonds in your favorite baked goods recipe to add a nutrition boost.

✔ Because about a quarter of the calories from almonds come from carbohydrates, they're made into almond flour. Use almond flour for gluten-free baking and cooking — in pancakes, cookies, muffins, and cake recipes.

✔ Ground almonds can be made into almond milk and used as a substitute for dairy. Use almond milk in your cereal, tea, or coffee, and instead of dairy in recipes.

✔ Almonds are ground into butter and used as a substitute for peanut butter with a sweeter taste. Use almond butter on whole wheat toast, spread it over fruit slices, add it to smoothies and oatmeal, and use it anywhere you'd use peanut butter.

If you're allergic to peanut butter, almond butter can be a helpful substitute.

✔ Almond paste or blanched almonds are used as a filling or addition to many Mediterranean pastries, cakes, and desserts. Bitter almonds are used in Italy as a base for cookies or macaroons.

Hazelnuts

Hazelnuts, also known as *filberts* and largely produced in Turkey, were one of the three nuts used in a large-scale Mediterranean diet study on heart health in 2013. The researchers used almonds, hazelnuts, and walnuts to show that the Mediterranean diet supplemented with nuts (one of the groups monitored) greatly reduces risk for coronary events and dying from heart disease.

Hazelnuts are a good source of B vitamins like thiamine and folate. These vitamins are essential for energy metabolism and cardiovascular health, and help create the hormone serotonin, which boosts your mood. They are also full of flavonoids like *proanthocyanidins*, which are the same kind of antioxidants that give green tea its benefits, including improving circulation and protecting brain health.

Although hazelnuts can be eaten raw or roasted, the nut and its oil are more frequently used to add a rich flavor to cookies, cakes, and chocolate recipes. They are also ground into flour for baking. You may be most familiar with hazelnuts as the main component of Nutella, which is made from roasted hazelnuts, skim milk, and cocoa.

The flavor of hazelnuts is more mellow and sweet when roasted. To roast hazelnuts, follow these steps:

1. **Remove the shell by using a nut cracker.**

2. **Place the nuts on a baking sheet and bake them on medium heat for 10 to 15 minutes.**

   You'll know they're done when the skin splits and kernels turn a golden color.

3. **Rub the skins off with a clean towel and enjoy!**

   Keep the roasted nuts refrigerated in an airtight container. Head to the later section "Storing and Preserving Nuts and Seeds" for more information on best methods for storing nuts.

Pine nuts

The popularity of pesto sauce has brought pine nuts into the American culinary spotlight in recent years. But this seed, originating from the pine tree, has been used for thousands of years.

In ancient Rome and Greece, pine nuts, or *pignoli,* were suggested to be an aphrodisiac, and today the Mediterranean pine nut crop comes specifically from a pine tree species in Spain, Portugal, and Italy. You can't just get pine nuts out of any pine cone that falls on the ground, but in certain areas and climates in America, they are produced with a sweet, fruity flavor that's tasty enough to eat.

The oil from pine nuts, *pinoleic acid*, is notable for studies suggesting that it triggers two hormones, including CCK (cholecystokinin), which help suppress your appetite and promote weight loss. Pine nuts are also a decent source of *lutein,* an antioxidant that's key to sharp vision and boosts your immune function.

Aside from using pine nuts in pesto sauce (comprised of pine nuts, basil, crushed garlic, olive oil, and Parmesan cheese) or topped on traditional Italian-American Pignoli cookies, you can also incorporate them in dishes by doing the following:

- ✔ Adding them to rice pilafs
- ✔ Sprinkling them over salads and vegetables
- ✔ Roasting them to add flavor to fish and meat dishes
- ✔ Baking them into breads and desserts
- ✔ Crushing them into other types of sauces and even grinding them into coffee

Pistachios

Pistachios can add a lot to your diet aside from just making a delicious ice cream or gelato flavor. Their antioxidant content, including vitamins A and E and lutein, has been shown to have a big beneficial impact beyond that found in a typical Mediterranean diet. A notable study published in the *Journal of Nutrition* in 2010 found that participants who included pistachios had higher blood levels of these antioxidants, which correlates to lower "bad" (LDL) cholesterol.

This green nut has a distinct crisp texture and sweet nutty flavor that's wonderful for snacking. Plus, aside from the health benefits that all nuts offer, pistachios give you a lot of bang for your caloric buck. One ounce of pistachios is about 47 kernels and around 170 calories. Because you have to take time to open and chew them, they increase satiation. Compare that to cashews (about 18 kernels of cashews for the same number of calories) or walnuts (about 14 walnut halves). In an ounce of pistachios, you'll also find the same amount of potassium you would in an orange.

Pistachios are found prominently in traditional desserts of the Mediterranean, like baklava, Turkish delight, and nougat. It was and is still frequently ground up for use in sauces or chopped and added to fruit or puddings.

If you're only eating pistachios as a snack and want to explore other ways of adding them to your diet immediately, try out some of these ideas:

- ✔ Add raw nuts to soups, salads, and grain dishes like barley or quinoa.
- ✔ Use crushed pistachios to coat fish, poultry, or tofu before baking.
- ✔ Blend pistachios into smoothies or shakes.
- ✔ Grind raw pistachios to add as a thickening agent to sauces or marinades.

Walnuts

Are walnuts the most nutritious nut? Researchers from the University of Scranton found that walnut's antioxidant content is almost double that of all other nuts, including almonds and hazelnuts.

In addition, unlike most nuts that contain primarily monounsaturated oils, walnuts are composed of mostly polyunsaturated omega-3 oils, and linoleic and alpha-linolenic acid. Therefore, walnuts have particular benefits in terms of reducing inflammation, risk of heart disease, and certain types of cancer. These omega-3 oils also benefit brain health and offer protection from cognitive decline (appropriate, don't you think, given that the walnut's shape resembles a brain?).

Although I can't definitively declare it as the best nut (because they all offer unique qualities, benefits, and uses), what is true is that walnuts are a staple of Mediterranean cuisine. Try to incorporate walnuts into your diet in the following ways:

- ✔ Tossed into salads, pastas, muesli, and yogurts
- ✔ Blended into salad dressings, marinades, and sauces (think walnut pesto!)
- ✔ Baked into breads and biscotti
- ✔ Toasted and sprinkled over poultry dishes
- ✔ Added to grains like couscous or bulgur pilaf for a nutty flavor
- ✔ Paired with dried fruit (like fig) or cheese (ricotta), and drizzled with honey for a treat
- ✔ Herbed or spiced for a kick with your snack

Sesame seeds

Most notably in Mediterranean cuisine, ground sesame seeds are used to make tahini. *Tahini* is a paste that is the major component of *hummus* (ground chickpeas), *baba ganoush* (eggplant-based dip), and *halva* (a popular confection).

Making your own tahini at home isn't too difficult. Follow these steps:

1. **Toast the sesame seeds for about 2 minutes in a pan, shaking every 15 seconds or so).**

2. **Mix the toasted seeds with olive oil (1 tablespoon for every ¼ cup seeds) in a blender until smooth.**

You may not consider that the seeds on your crackers, breads, and bun would be chockfull of nutrition benefits. But sesame actually contains more calcium than any other nut or seed (the amount even increases when the seed is toasted). Just a quarter cup of sesame seeds gives you the same amount of calcium as a glass of milk.

Think outside the hamburger bun! Sesame seeds can be incorporated in salads, added to stir-fries, included on sushi rolls, mashed into condiments and spreads, and used in a variety of sauces and marinades.

Integrating This Winning Combo into Mediterranean Fare

Whether nuts, seeds, and legumes are the main event of a Mediterranean meal or a part of a snack or side dish, they'll certainly complement your diet with a variety of nutrients and flavor. In this section, you discover how these foods fit in with traditional Mediterranean fare and how to use them as a substitute for foods you're currently eating. You'll also find out the right amount of servings to have each day. After all, you can have too much of a good thing.

Saying "Nuts!" to a low-fat diet: Including nuts and seeds in your diet

Nuts and seeds are just one of the heart-healthy sources of fat encouraged on the Mediterranean diet (the other two are fatty fish, covered in Chapter 12, and olive oil, covered in Chapter 8).

When you add nuts, seeds, and legumes into your Mediterranean diet, you can use them to replace other sources of calories you currently consume from artery-clogging saturated fat and refined carbohydrates. Table 9-1 gives you an idea of how your diet can be augmented for the better with nuts, seeds, and beans. This guide can help you improve your nutrient profile at various meals by reducing your intake of saturated fats and giving you more fiber. Use these substitutions as inspiration as you try to think of other ways to swap out less healthy ingredients for more healthy fare.

Table 9-1	A Guide to Swapping in Nuts, Seeds, Legumes	
Instead of This	*Choose This*	*Nutrition Wins*
Egg and cheese sandwich	Peanut butter sandwich	Lose 5 grams saturated fat Gain 2 grams fiber
Chicken noodle soup	Lentil soup	Gain 6 grams fiber
Caesar salad	Walnut and cranberry salad	Lose 5 grams saturated fat Gain 10 grams fiber
Chicken cutlet	Pistachio crusted salmon	Lose 3 grams saturated fat Gain 2 grams fiber
Mushroom risotto	Almond rice pilaf	Lose 5 grams saturated fat Gain 3 grams fiber

Just like olive oil (Chapter 8), nuts and seeds are nutrient-dense: They give you a lot of nutrition in a small package. Although that is positive in many regards, it can also backfire if you don't keep your portions in check. Even if you are eating only nutritious foods but eating portions that are too large or eating too many servings, you can ingest too many calories and gain weight. Going overboard with nuts and seeds is easy because they're so small, and the calories add up quickly.

When eating nuts and seeds, as a general rule, stick to 1 ounce per day, every day. Instead of eating directly out of a large container or mindlessly pouring nuts or seeds into a recipe, always portion out a serving for yourself. Table 9-2 shows what an ounce of some favorite varieties gives you quantity-wise.

Table 9-2	Quantities per Ounce of Nuts and Seeds		
Nut	**Quantity**	**Calories**	**Fat (grams)**
Pistachios	49 kernels	160	13
Almond	23 nuts	160	14
Sesame seeds	2 tablespoons	160	14
Hazelnuts	21 kernels	178	17
Walnuts	14 halves	185	18.5
Pine nuts	167 kernels	190	19

Source: Based on the USDA Nutrient Database

Adding legumes to your diet

Legumes are a great source of both protein and fiber, two nutrients that contribute to feeling satiated. (The full feeling lasts longer with protein and fiber because these two nutrients take the longest for your body to digest.) Legumes can also be a substitute for higher-in-saturated-fat proteins like meat or full-fat dairy. They can also be a substitute for starches, like refined grains.

You can't really go wrong with any type of legume you add, from black beans to soy to lentil to cannellini (white kidney beans). Here are some Mediterranean favorites you can easily try at home:

✔ Puree chickpeas and tahini into hummus for sandwiches or dip.

✔ Add lentils to any type of salad, hot or cold.

✔ Cook cannellini beans with chard, escarole, or spinach.

🖊 Add black beans to grain dishes, like quinoa or barley

🖊 Add cooked kidney beans to an omelet.

🖊 Make chili with a variety of legumes — any type you enjoy!

Most dried beans and peas, except for black-eyed peas and lentils, require soaking in water before cooking. For guidance on cooking beans, head to Chapter 14.

Storing and Preserving Nuts and Seeds

You don't need to be a squirrel to understand the value of storing and preserving nuts and seeds. One of the fantastic traits of these foods is that they can last for a while without much hassle, allowing you to stock your kitchen with healthy options to grab and go. But if you've bought in bulk before, you may have been victim to rancid nuts and seeds as you check your store a few weeks after purchase.

So what's the best way to extend their shelf-life, you ask? Read on:

🖊 **Keep them in airtight, non-permeable containers.** Ditch the plastic bag and twist ties. Use glass jars instead. Nuts and seeds absorb odors from the outside if in permeable packaging, and air contributes to rancidness. If you can't use glass containers (like when you're freezing them; see later in this list), double up on plastic bags.

🖊 **Keep them in a dry, cool, dark place.** A pantry that doesn't get much light works (if you plan to eat them within 2 to 4 months), but the refrigerator or freezer is best. Refrigerated or frozen, they keep for longer (between 1 to 2 years).

Moisture, heat, and light are enemies to freshness of nuts and seeds because they oxidize the nuts' and seeds' natural oils.

🖊 **Buy whole, raw nuts.** Chopped, sliced, and blanched nuts don't last as long as whole nuts and seeds, so if you have the option, depending on how you consume the nuts, go for the unprocessed varieties.

Because they are more easily broken down, unsaturated fats found in nuts, seeds, and oils turn rancid more quickly than saturated fats. When oxidized, they're more likely to taste and smell bad, so you should be able to identify when they've gone sour. As they say, "When it doubt, throw it out."

Chapter 10

Fruits and Veggies: Key Parts of This Plant-Based Diet

. . . .

In This Chapter

▶ Discovering the benefits of nature's fruits and vegetables

▶ Understanding what varieties are all-stars of the Mediterranean diet

▶ Knowing how much you need and how to get those servings in

. . . .

As you may expect, a plant-based diet such as the Mediterranean diet would be chockfull of nature's candy — fruits and vegetables! It's probably not a complete shock that they should be a key part of your diet because you've heard it before: from the USDA telling you that half your plate should contain them, from fruit- and veggie-filled products touting their nutritional benefits, and from the media releasing research studies about those benefits and their link to weight loss or disease prevention.

Unfortunately, even with all of this knowledge and on top of the desire to eat more healthfully (according to survey responses), Americans are still not getting enough fruits and vegetables.

Eating enough does more than just add color to your plate; it also fills you up with nutrients like antioxidants, vitamins, minerals, and fiber. Because each type offers unique health perks, the more variety, the better. This chapter tells you about the variety of fruits and vegetables within the Mediterranean diet, explains how many servings you need daily, and offers advice on how to start incorporating those foods into your diet today.

Even though it's not always easy being green and the reasons for not getting your dose of fruits and veggies are complex, this chapter explains how getting your fill can be the first step of a seamless transition to a more nutritious, Mediterranean diet.

Eating Local: An Overview of Mediterranean Produce

Including fruits and vegetables at every meal comes naturally in the Mediterranean lifestyle, and soon enough, it'll be second nature for you, too! One reason the people of Mediterranean countries eat so much fruit and vegetables is that they eat food grown in their own backyards, and many varieties of fruits and vegetables flourish in the Mediterranean climate.

Eating foods — especially produce — grown as close to home as possible maximizes the nutrition you get out of them. Why? Because nutrient concentration begins to decrease after harvesting. The more time that passes between harvest and consumption, the fewer nutrients there are. During transportation, when foods are handled or processed, the nutrients (and taste) decline. Choosing local, in-season produce provides the best nutrition, the best taste, and the best cost, too.

Countries of the Mediterranean like Italy, Greece, and Spain enjoy at home and export their most popular fruit and vegetables, which include

- **Fruits:** Apricots, avocado, cherries, citrus, figs, olives, peaches, pomegranates
- **Vegetables:** Artichokes, eggplants, onions, sweet potatoes, zucchini

Later in this chapter, I delve more deeply into many of these varieties and point out their specific benefits, as well as the best ways to include them in your diet. For now, remember that how you eat your fruits and veggies is just as important as how many servings of them you get daily. In American diets, fruits and veggies are often part of dishes with refined sugars or served breaded and fried. In the Mediterranean, on the other hand, vegetables can be eaten raw for breakfast, and fresh fruit is often the basis for dessert. Even if you're already eating plenty of fruits and veggies, following the Mediterranean diet will help you change the way you eat them for the better.

Understanding the Benefits of Fruits and Veggies

Instead of blindly following advice to get between seven and ten servings of fruits and veggies every day (people in the Mediterranean get an average of nine servings per day!), it's important to understand the benefits of filling half of your plate with colorful fruits and vegetables.

The color is not just for show. Each color of fruit and veggie, from red beets to orange carrots to white cauliflower, represents phytonutrients that give the fruit or veggie health benefits. By eating from the rainbow, you get a mix of antioxidants that help fight disease like heart disease and cancer, protect your immune function, and improve your brain function. In addition, fruits and vegetables contain the following:

- ✔ **Fiber.** All fruits and vegetables contain fiber, which helps reduce cholesterol, lower blood pressure, and improve digestive health. Fiber can also reduce your risk for some types of cancers. In addition, foods with fiber fill you up and keep you more satisfied. Research shows that people who meet their fiber needs (at least 25 grams per day for women, 38 grams per day for men) are more likely to lose weight and keep it off.

- ✔ **Potassium.** This mineral helps reduce high blood pressure and plays a role in normal brain function. If you've had cramps, you may have been told to eat a banana; that's because the potassium is key for normal muscle contraction. Potassium is also dense in tomatoes, potatoes, and leafy green veggies.

- ✔ **Vitamin A.** The orange color of carrots, oranges, and apricots is due to the presence of beta-carotene, which is converted into vitamin A in your body. Ever hear carrots are good for your eyes? That's because vitamin A helps protect eye health; it also works as an immune booster.

- ✔ **Vitamin C.** You can get a solid dose of vitamin C from oranges, red and green peppers, strawberries, sweet potatoes, and broccoli, to name a few items. Although it's not a cure for the common cold, vitamin C can help reduce your risk for infection. People who eat more vitamin C have higher levels of the vitamin in their blood, and at least one study in the *American Journal of Clinical Nutrition* associated these higher levels with a much lower risk for stroke. Vitamin C is also an antioxidant, protecting your cells inside and outside, and it can help reduce signs of aging.

- ✔ **Folate.** This B vitamin is key for cell repair and brain function. All prenatal vitamins contain folate because it's vital for fetal brain and spinal cord development. You find folate in green leafy vegetables, like spinach, kale, and broccoli, as well as in strawberries and oranges. Folate helps remove *homocysteine,* a compound that can cause artery damage, so it's important for heart health and can reduce your risk for stroke.

Two other obvious benefits that still merit being stated: 1) When you eat fruits and vegetables at every single meal or snack, you're eating fewer items that may not be as nutritious. 2) The fiber and high water content of many fruits and vegetables allow you to eat larger portions for fewer calories than most foods. As a bonus, not only are you getting more nutrition, but you'll also be more satisfied and better able to keep your portions in check throughout the day.

If you're thinking the message of this section is that the good vegetables do for you makes up for their taste, let me disabuse you of that notion. Fruits and vegetables can be delicious, and I show you how in the remaining sections of this chapter!

Zoning In on the Top Mediterranean Fruits

There's more to fruit than just apples and bananas, delicious as those are. If you tend to choose the same traditional fruits over and over, the most popular fruits of the Mediterranean cuisine will certainly broaden your fruit horizon and give you new flavors, textures, and health benefits. Who knows? Maybe the new saying will be that a pomegranate a day keeps the doctor away!

Avocados

When I was growing up, avocados were reserved for guacamole paired with tortilla chips on Super Bowl Sunday. Now, this pear-shaped green fruit with a leather-like skin is everywhere and used in a variety of dishes. Although this fruit is very widespread and versatile, where it can grow is not. Avocados can be cultivated only in tropical or Mediterranean climates and sometimes in more temperate climates like California.

Avocados aren't your typical fruit. Their flavor isn't sweet or their texture crisp. Instead, avocados have a smooth, creamy, and rich texture due to the presence of fat — which is also absent from most fruit varieties. Because of this, avocados have a unique place in your diet. Here are some things to know:

- They're often added in lieu of meat for vegetarian dishes. They're a rare source of both heart-healthy fat and fiber. (Nuts and seeds do the same, so if you are allergic to those, avocados can be an excellent substitute for you.) Try the following:

  - Slice them up and add them to salads (use avocados in a sweet fruit salad for variety).

  - Top sandwiches or burgers with them.

  - Blend them into smoothies.

  - Scramble them into eggs.

  - Eat them straight up!

- Most of the calories you consume with avocados come from the polyunsaturated omega-3 fatty acids and monounsaturated fatty acids (*oleic acid,* the same fat found in olive oil) within. These fatty acids act to lower "bad" (LDL) cholesterol and raise "good" (HDL) cholesterol. The remaining calories in avocados come from heart-healthy and cancer-fighting fiber.

- Because they are rich in fat, they are calorie- and nutrient-dense. Just 1 ounce (or about one-fifth of a medium avocado) gives you about 50 calories, 5 grams of fat, 3 grams of fiber, and dozens of vitamins, minerals, and phytonutrients like potassium, B vitamins, vitamin C, vitamin E, and *lutein,* an antioxidant that protects eye health and prevents macular degeneration.

Avocados, like bananas, mature on the tree, but they don't ripen until they've been picked. That's why avocados are found rock-hard at the store. You know they are ripe and ready to eat when the skin yields to gentle pressure. You can refrigerate them to slow the ripening process. After you peel or cut one open, add lemon or lime juice to prevent browning.

Avocados are best eaten raw. Avoid heating avocados too much; doing so releases bitter chemicals that impact their natural taste.

Figs

Figs are one of the first plants that humans cultivated to eat. Not only are they traditional in Mediterranean cuisine, but they are in ever-increasing demand around the world. These small, sweet, pear-shaped fruits with the edible seeds have a thin and fuzzy skin that is often purple or brown when ripened.

Figs are often dried or preserved in jams, because fresh figs are very delicate and don't last long at room temperature. These are also the reasons that figs don't travel well. Because they are so perishable, if you buy them fresh, keep them refrigerated and eat them within a couple of days.

Figs develop from a cluster of flowers on the fig tree after being pollinated by a special fig wasp. In Ancient Greece, dried figs were a major part of the diet for both rich and poor, and they were actually consumed by Olympians to improve stamina and speed. This practice was likely due to the high sugar content of the dried fruit and its fiber content, which helps keep you satisfied and energized!

Figs, whether fresh or dried, can be a sweet addition to any diet; they also add Mediterranean flair to dishes:

- ✔ Add figs to a salad with walnuts and shaved Parmesan
- ✔ Poach figs in red wine and serve with low-fat Greek yogurt
- ✔ Make a grain salad, like quinoa, with figs and veggies
- ✔ Stuff fresh figs with cheese and nut slivers as an appetizer
- ✔ Place figs on top of crostini and pizza, and in sandwiches
- ✔ Serve them alone as a dessert
- ✔ Chop dried figs into oatmeal and top with cinnamon

Figs have a natural laxative effect because of their high fiber content. If you need to add fiber to your diet or want to relieve constipation, try figs!

Mandarins

You may only recognize the term *mandarin* from canned mandarin oranges, but chances are you've also consumed a mandarin in its fresh form, too. In America, the most common type of mandarin orange is the tangerine, originally exported from the city of Tangiers in Morocco. Clementine is another variety of mandarin you may be familiar with. Over the past few decades, mandarin production has increased considerably in the Mediterranean in places like Spain and Italy. (The term *mandarin* applies to a wide range of citrus fruit that has a thin, easy-to-peel skin and easy-to-eat segments, either seeded or seedless.)

Mandarins are a great food to eat solo. Just one small mandarin orange has 37 calories and can contain 30 percent of your vitamin C and 10 percent of your vitamin A needs for the day! Seedless varieties are a great way to get your child to eat fruit, because they're fun and easy to eat. You can also try slicing them up into salads, stir fries, yogurts, and desserts, or including them as part of a marinade or a stuffing for poultry dishes.

Store a crate of tangerines or other mandarins in the refrigerator for up to two weeks.

Olives

The Mediterranean cultivates about 95 percent of the world's olives, which are eaten as a fruit or pressed for their oil. (To find out how olive oil is made from this valuable commodity and its prominent place in the Mediterranean diet, refer to Chapter 8.)

Because of their heart-healthy fat content, olives, like avocados, don't have the sweet flavor you'd expect from something called a fruit. Green olives are picked before they're ripe and, therefore, have a more bitter flavor than the brown or black olives, which stay on the tree longer, do. Raw olives also must be cured in brine before being eaten, and this can give them a salty flavor.

Traditionally, olives are served on the table in olive oil before a meal, added as a garnish to cocktails, stuffed with cheese, sliced atop pizzas and salads, cooked with fish, and so on. If you're adding olives to a hot dish, toss them in at the last minute. Exposure to heat makes them even more bitter. Store opened jars of olives in your refrigerator and follow the "Use By" date on the jar for freshness.

Many varieties of olives are available. Some of the most popular olives include

- ✔ **Kalamata:** This is a popular Greek black olive with a fruitier flavor than other olives.

- ✔ **Manzanilla:** These large, green Spanish olives are usually pitted and stuffed with pimento. You'll usually see them in a martini glass.

- ✔ **Gaeta:** This small, black, Italian olive is wrinkled, often packed in oil, and has a meaty texture.

Pomegranates

Although pomegranates are native to Persia and heralded as the oldest known edible fruit, pomegranate trees have been cultivated by many Mediterranean countries and grown commercially throughout the world. In the past several years, pomegranates have been touted as super foods in America and for good reason.

Pomegranates are rich in polyphenols called *punicalagins,* which are powerful antioxidants that can reduce cholesterol and blood pressure as well as improve arterial health.

Eating a pomegranate may seem intimidating, not to mention messy. After all, only the juice and seeds inside the tough outer layer are edible. But their delicious taste and health benefits are well worth it. Pomegranate juice adds a natural red food coloring to beverages, and the seeds can make a wonderful addition to salads, sprinkled over desserts, or served with olives (thus pairing sweet and salty flavors).

To keep your clothes and kitchen stain-free, follow these steps to get through the rind and to the seeds and juice:

1. **Cut off and discard the crown end of the pomegranate.**

   Just cut far enough to see the seeds within.

2. **Using a sharp knife, cut through just the peel (not completely through the fruit) from stem to end in several sections.**

3. **Pull apart the sections and peel off pieces of white membranes and push the sections out over a bowl so the seeds fall out.**

   Ripe seeds will fall off easily, but you may have to gently rub off the others with your fingers.

Many suggest performing this step with the pomegranate submerged in a bowl of cold water to reduce the mess. If you do so, the seeds fall to the bottom of the bowl and the rest (like the membrane) floats to the top. Simply skim the floating stuff from the water and strain the seeds.

Each medium pomegranate will yield about one cup of seeds.

To make juice, place your seeds in a blender and pulse a couple of times so the seeds release their juice. Pour the chunky mixture into a mesh strainer over a bowl. Using the back of a spoon, push as much of the pulp through the strainer as you can. Add sugar or natural sweetener to taste and add water until you reach the consistency you desire. Drink the juice straight up or add it to smoothies or cocktails.

Zoning In on the Top Mediterranean Vegetables

Although adding more vegetables in general to your diet is inherently more Mediterranean, certain vegetables stand out as key components of a Mediterranean diet. In this section, I focus on the top five Mediterranean veggies and explain what they do for your health and diet.

Artichokes

The artichoke plant, or globe artichoke, is native to the Mediterranean region and cultivated primarily in countries like France, Italy, Spain, and Morocco. A story from Greek mythology says that Zeus turned a woman he loved but who betrayed him into the first artichoke as punishment — a story that makes perfect sense when you consider that an artichoke is a rather thorny plant with a hard exterior.

Although only a small portion of the artichoke is eaten, it ranks number one in antioxidants compared to any other vegetable, according to the USDA. Also, if you eat all the edible parts of a medium-sized artichoke, you get about 10 grams of fiber (about one-third of your daily needs) and a good dose of vitamin C in just 64 calories.

How exactly and what parts are you supposed to eat of this tough vegetable? Read on:

✔ You can boil or steam the veggie whole (after removing the stem and spiky tops) and break off the outer petals one by one, dunk them into sauce or dip, and eat the tender part at the bottom of each petal.

To extract the soft interior from the hard exterior petal (which is not edible), simply pull the petal slowly between your front teeth. This maneuver is similar to the one you use to eat edamame.

✔ You can eat the artichoke heart after removing the inedible fuzzy part that covers it. Artichoke hearts are typically used in cooking and added to many Mediterranean favorites. Here are some suggestions:

- Chop up the heart and include it in Mediterranean tuna salad along with olives, spices, and herbs.

- Add the heart to a traditional Italian *minestra* soup, along with white beans.

- Toss the heart in with seafood-based pastas.

- Grill artichoke hearts and add them to an antipasto salad or serve them as a side dish.

- Make a chopped artichoke-and-spinach dip with low-fat cheese or yogurt.

- Stuff artichokes with whole wheat bread crumbs, pine nuts, and herbs.

Eggplant

When many people think about eggplant, they automatically think eggplant Parmesan, a dish that smothers all the nutrition of eggplant in a fried concoction featuring breadcrumbs and mozzarella cheese. But this purple veggie on its own contains only about 20 calories per cooked cup, 2.5 grams of fiber, and *anthocyanins,* the antioxidants that give eggplant its purple hue.

Not only do these antioxidants have heart health and cancer fighting properties, but preliminary research in rats published in the *Journal of Agricultural and Food Chemistry* in 2010 also found that anthocyanins may offer protection against obesity and diabetes.

The entire eggplant, including purple skin and white flesh, is edible and tastes best when cooked (the raw fruit has a bitter taste). Eggplant tends to soak up a lot of oil in dishes, so be extra aware of your portions, especially when you're dining out and can't control how much olive oil is added to the dish.

Just because it's a vegetable doesn't mean the eggplant can't be the main show. Due to its fleshy skin, eggplant can act as a meat substitute and is the star of many Mediterranean dishes:

✔ **Baba ganoush:** Popular in Turkey, this appetizer is made with eggplant, olive oil, and herbs.

✔ **Moussaka:** Greece and Turkey each have their own variations of this dish, but both are essentially eggplant casseroles, either baked or sautéed. Moussaka can include minced meat (use a lean cut of meat or turkey), potatoes, peppers, tomatoes, zucchini, and other veggies.

- ✓ **Eggplant Parmesan or rollatini:** Make a baked version with whole wheat breadcrumbs and go light on the cheese (and/or choose low-fat cheese) to save on calories and fat.
- ✓ **Topping for pizza or pasta:** Instead of using meat toppings, add baked eggplant to your pizza, or add diced eggplant to a pasta dish.
- ✓ **Eggplant chips or "fries":** Instead of potatoes, bake eggplant slices or sticks with herbs, spices, and whole wheat bread crumbs.

Onions

If you equate dark, vibrant fruit and vegetable colors with healthy properties, you may mistakenly think that onions (especially white onions) are devoid of nutrition. But much research has been conducted on the allium family — onions, garlic, scallions — and the antioxidants or allyl sulfides they contain may be one reason for lower cancer rates among people who consume large quantities of these veggies.

Although they may not be great for your breath, onions also have antibacterial properties that help you fight infections, compounds to help lower blood pressure, and *chromium,* a mineral that may be helpful in keeping your blood glucose in check.

Maybe it's no surprise that the Mediterranean people consume copious amounts of onions and garlic (Chapter 17 has for more on garlic). You can add onions to salads, grains, fish or poultry, dips and spreads — anything you eat!

Wear goggles when chopping onions! You'll look silly, but the goggles will help prevent you from tearing up. When chopping onions, a compound called *sulfenic acid* is released, which irritates the eyes and causes tearing. Chopping in a well-ventilated area or with a fan blowing may also help lessen the effect.

Sweet potatoes

How sweet it is to get a dose of fiber, potassium, vitamin A, and vitamin C in something as delicious as a sweet potato! You may be familiar with sweet potatoes — made into sweet potato fries, mashed at Thanksgiving (yams are actually a different veggie altogether), or baked with a pat of butter. But how do the Mediterranean people do sweet potatoes? They enjoy them in the following dishes, to name just a few:

- ✓ Sweet potato soup
- ✓ Sweet potato Spanish tortilla
- ✓ Sweet potato gnocchi

✔ Sweet potato cake

✔ Sweet potato frittata

Any way you eat white potatoes, you can substitute sweet potatoes, which offer a better nutrient profile. But remember this tip: Don't peel your potatoes! A lot of the nutrition, including the belly-filling and heart-disease–fighting fiber, is found in the skin. Also, pair sweet potatoes with a source of fat, like drizzled olive oil or chopped nuts, to help your body absorb the beta-carotene.

Zucchini

Zucca is the Italian word for squash, and zucchini, a type of summer squash, was developed and is still heavily used in Italian cuisine. Zucchini contains fiber and many vitamins inherent in other veggies but is also a good source of manganese. This mineral is helpful for energy metabolism, breaking down and helping your body use carbohydrates and protein.

Whereas the extent of your zucchini knowledge may lie in fried zucchini sticks, in the Mediterranean countries, zucchini is used in a variety of dishes, like zucchini bread, zucchini pancakes, dips and spreads, and toppings for salads and sandwiches.

One great way to eat zucchini is in strips as a substitute for pasta. Alternatively, you can add it to pasta dishes to bulk up the nutritional value.

Striving for Health with Seven to Ten Servings

Consuming seven to ten servings of fruits and vegetables a day may seem like a lot, but it doesn't have to be such a challenge. The next sections offer all sorts of suggestions.

If you don't love the fruits and veggies specifically associated with the Mediterranean diet, that's okay! Eat any type of fruit or vegetable you like — and the more the merrier. The later section "Enjoying a rainbow of alternatives" offers a variety of options to choose from.

Research shows an inverse relationship between number of fruits and veggies and the risk for disease: The more fruits and vegetables you eat, the less likely you are to get sick. Between seven and ten servings seems to be the range for the biggest reductions in disease risk. So how can you meet that lucky number of servings? Read on.

Sneaking fruits and veggies into every meal

At every single meal and snack, choose at least a serving or two (or three!) of a fruit or vegetable. Do so not only for the nutrients and the taste, but also to help round out every meal and keep you satisfied with fiber.

What is a serving? This table shows you:

Food	Serving Size
Fresh fruit	½ cup
Dried fruit	¼ cup
raw vegetables	1 cup
Cooked vegetables	½ cup

But if you don't want to remember these stats, as an overarching guideline, simply aim for 2 to 3 cups of fruit and 2 to 3 cups of veggies every day.

When you're planning ahead, ask yourself, "What is my fruit or vegetable at this meal?" If the answer is nothing, and you need (or your picky child needs) to get a dose, refer to Table 10-1, which highlights some sneaky ways to integrate fruits and vegetables at breakfast, lunch, and dinner!

Table 10-1	Sneaking in a Dose of Fruits and Vegetables at Every Meal
Meal	*Fruit and Veggie Suggestions*
Breakfast	Make a fruit and/or veggie-packed smoothie.
	Use canned pumpkin in your muffins.
	Add pureed banana in your pancakes.
Lunch	Add a slice of avocado or onions to your sandwich.
	Chop up spinach into soups or as topping for pizza.
Dinner	Make zucchini pancakes or figs with walnuts for an appetizer.
	Top a chicken or fish with mango salsa.
	Use spaghetti squash in place of pasta.

Enjoying a rainbow of alternatives

Eating from the rainbow of hues ensure you get a variety of nutrients and keeps you from getting bored with your selections. (If you're not so keen on the most popular Mediterranean fruits and veggies, you can try some of the these on for size!):

- ✓ **Red:** Apples, beets, cherries, cranberries, raspberries, strawberries, tomatoes
- ✓ **Orange/yellow:** Apricots, butternut squash, cantaloupe, carrots, peaches, pumpkin
- ✓ **Green:** Asparagus, broccoli, Brussels sprouts, kale, spinach
- ✓ **Blue/Purple:** Blackberries, blueberries, grapes, plums
- ✓ **White:** Bananas, cauliflower, jicama, mushrooms

Swapping in fruit for dessert

When you hear the word *dessert,* your mind may wander to thoughts of cookies, cake, and ice cream. Although those foods are okay to have once in a while, they shouldn't be everyday indulgences. If you have a sweet tooth, you may find that swapping in fruit can help give you the sweet satisfaction you need while helping you consume less of the more indulgent stuff. So do like people in the Mediterranean region do and swap in these delicious and more nutritious dessert ideas:

- ✓ Fresh berry sorbet
- ✓ Sliced peaches soaked in wine
- ✓ Halved figs with a drizzle of honey
- ✓ Baked apples or pears
- ✓ Greek yogurt with dried apricots

Everything in moderation! If you want to have cookies or cake once in a while, that's fine. In fact, indulging periodically is also the Mediterranean way. Fruit tarts and cakes are popular dishes. As long as you keep your portions in check and make these treats an occasional — and not an everyday — thing they can be part of a healthful diet.

Going organic, fresh, or frozen

Two questions that I get asked frequently may very well be on your mind, too:

"Do I need to buy organic fruits and veggies?"

"Are frozen fruits and veggies just as good as fresh?"

The short answers, in order, are "Not always" and "Yes."

Organic fruits and vegetables are not necessarily nutritionally superior, but they are grown without synthetic fertilizers or pesticides. The additional cost to the farm for using more environmentally friendly practices and manpower are transferred to you, the consumer. Although no definitive research proves that the chemicals used in conventional farming are bad for your health, they are still synthetic chemicals, which have the potential to be harmful.

The Environmental Working Group (EWG), a health advocacy and research group, puts certain fruits and veggies on its "Dirty Dozen" list, meaning they're the ones that absorb the most chemicals. If you're going to spend the extra cost on organic, choose these items. Out of the Mediterranean favorites, only potatoes are on the dirty list whereas onions and avocados are on the EWG's cleanest list. For more, visit http://www.ewg.org/.

When choosing between fresh and frozen, feel free to choose frozen to save money and get your favorite fruits and veggies out of season. Typically frozen at the peak of ripeness, frozen fruits and veggies can retain more nutrients than fresh ones that deal with traveling and handling.

Chapter 11

Great Grains

Comparing Whole to Refined Grains

In This Chapter

▶ Getting familiar with the benefits of whole versus refined grains

▶ Identifying the grain all-stars of the Mediterranean diet

▶ Understanding how to incorporate grains and navigate common allergies

*O*ver the past decade, grains popularized in Mediterranean cuisine have entered the spotlight as super foods. Some of these grains are called "ancient" because they've been around for thousands of years and have remained unchanged. In the food industry business, grains that are processed after harvest are stripped of their wholesome nutrition. Unfortunately, you're probably eating too many of these refined grains because they're so easy and cheap to produce, and they make up the bulk of what's available on store shelves. In this chapter, you discover the differences between whole (and wholesome!) grains and why choosing whole grains provides more healthy benefits.

As you embark on your Mediterranean lifestyle and reduce your consumption of refined grains, you'll begin to expand your grain horizons beyond breads and rice dishes. When grains common in the Mediterranean also become common in your kitchen, you'll not only reap health benefits but will also benefit from greater taste and more variety in your diet. Grains, from bulgur to quinoa, are extremely versatile and pair perfectly with many flavors, keeping your stomach and your taste buds satisfied.

Don't be surprised or intimidated if you've never eaten some of the grains mentioned in this chapter. I outline quick and easy ways to incorporate them. You can also head to Chapter 16, which includes recipes that include some of these grains.

If you or someone you know suffers from a wheat and/or gluten allergy, keep reading. I've included advice in here to help you navigate through the various options so that you know which grains to choose and which to avoid while still coming out on top nutrition-wise!

Comparing Whole Grains to Refined Grains

If the extent of your knowledge on this topic begins and ends with the fact that whole grain bread is brown and refined grain bread is white, get ready to embark on a journey of discover! This section gives you the lowdown on what whole grains are, what happens when they're refined, and how nutrients and health benefits differ in each.

Before diving in, it'll help you to know what a grain is, exactly. According to the USDA, any food that is made from wheat, rice, oats, cornmeal, barley, or another cereal grain falls into the grains category. Any of these grains can be eaten in their whole or refined form, but they all start out as whole grains.

The whole truth and nothing but the truth: Whole grains

When something is "whole," it has all of its parts. And the same is true with whole grains. When grown, whole grains contain the entire seed of the plant, which consists of three main, edible sections (see Figure 11-1):

✔ **Endosperm:** Making up the largest part of the kernel, the endosperm is the germ's food supply. It contains mostly carbohydrate and smaller amounts of protein, vitamins, and minerals.

✔ **Germ:** The *germ* is the embryo, fed by the endosperm, which can sprout into a new plant. The germ contains B vitamins and a small amount of protein, fat, and minerals.

✔ **Bran:** As the outer layer of the kernel, the bran contains fiber, antioxidants, and B vitamins.

Unfortunately only about 10 to 15 percent of the products in a typical American grocery store are 100 percent whole grain (that is, containing the bran, germ, and endosperm). Don't be deceived by labels that say "multigrain" or "made with whole grain." Make sure the label reads, "100 percent whole grain." That way, you know you're getting the real deal.

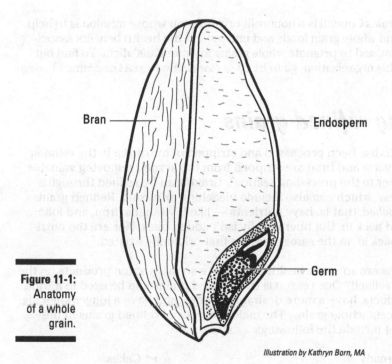

Bran —

Endosperm

Germ

Figure 11-1:
Anatomy
of a whole
grain.

Illustration by Kathryn Born, MA

Here are some examples of whole grain products to look for:

- Bulgur
- Barley
- Buckwheat
- Farro
- Freekah
- Oats or oatmeal

- Quinoa
- Brown or wild rice
- Popcorn
- Wheat berries
- Whole grain flour

Because many foods contain a mixture of grains, make sure your product contains at least some whole grains. Check the list of ingredients. One of the first ingredients should read "whole wheat" or "whole grain." (**Note:** Ideally you want that phrase to be close to the top of the ingredient list because ingredients are listed on food labels by weight.) In addition to checking the ingredients, also look for a Whole Grains Council stamp on the package (although not all products that are whole grain will contain it).

The Whole Grains Council is a nonprofit organization whose mission is to help consumers find whole grain foods and understand the health benefits associated with them, and to promote whole grains in Americans' diets. To find out more about this organization, go to http://www.wholegrainscouncil.org.

Exposing refined grains

A *refined* grain has been processed and stripped of nutrition. In the refining process, the germ and bran are stripped from the kernel, removing valuable nutrients (refer to the preceding section). Grains can be refined through a milling process, which can also include bleaching or mixing. Refined grains are often *enriched,* that is, have nutrients — like B vitamins, iron, and folic acid — added back in. But fiber usually isn't added back. Nor are the nutrients added back in, in the same amounts that originally existed.

If whole grains are so much healthier, why are so many grain products on the marketplace refined? One reason is that refined grains can be used in a wide range of products, have a more desirable texture, and have a longer shelf life over 100 percent whole grains. The major sources of refined grains in the American diet include the following:

- White breads
- White rice
- Pastas
- Tortillas
- Taco shells
- Pizza dough
- Cakes
- Cookies
- Pies
- Pastries
- Potato chips
- Pretzels

One major problem with refined grains is that they are often found in products that also contain saturated fat, sodium, and additives. If your diet is comprised mainly of these items, then it's time to Mediterranean-*ize* it!

Exploring the Benefits of Whole Grains

Going whole grain is a large component of the more locally sourced, less-processed Mediterranean diet. Your body needs carbohydrates from grains for energy, and it can use both refined or whole as an energy source. But as you start to reduce the refined grains you eat and swap in whole grains from foods like whole wheat pasta to polenta, you'll reap both natural nutrient and taste benefits, as the next sections explain.

How much is enough? Well, the more of your refined grains you swap out for whole, the better! At the very minimum, have one serving of whole grain at every meal to meet your nutritional needs. One serving is about an ounce (the equivalent of one slice of bread or a half cup of cooked grain). Research shows that eating whole grains, as little as one to three servings per day, has clear health benefits:

- ✔ Reduced heart disease risk
- ✔ Reduced stroke risk
- ✔ Normalized blood pressure levels
- ✔ Reduced risk for type 2 diabetes
- ✔ Improved weight loss and maintenance

So ditch the all-or-nothing mentality when it comes to adding whole grains. Every little bit counts toward a healthier you!

Focusing on fiber

Americans are only meeting about half their fiber needs. With whole grains, you typically get more fiber, which has plenty of health benefits:

- ✔ It reduces risk for high cholesterol, high blood pressure, and some types of cancer, and improves digestion.
- ✔ High-fiber foods make you feel fuller on fewer calories, which can help you keep your weight in check.
- ✔ Because fiber isn't digested or as easily broken down as refined carbs are, you have better blood glucose control, which positively impacts your body's insulin mechanism and your food cravings.

As you add more whole grains containing fiber to your diet, do so slowly. Add one additional serving every couple of days. Also, make sure you're drinking enough fluids, which helps process the fiber through your digestive tract. If you're constipated as you meet your fiber needs (25 grams for women, 38 grams for men per day), you probably aren't drinking enough.

Fiber is found not only in whole grains but also in fruits, veggies, nuts, and seeds (refer to Chapters 9 and 10 for more on those food groups).

Two main types of fiber are found in the diet, and neither is more important than the other. In addition, both types appear in all foods, but in different proportions, so it's good to have a mix of both:

✔ **Soluble fiber:** This type of fiber dissolves in water and forms a gel in your digestive tract which helps slow the movement of food. It's beneficial for stabilizing your blood glucose levels and reducing your "bad" (LDL) cholesterol levels.

✔ **Insoluble fiber:** Insoluble fiber doesn't dissolve in water. It provides bulk and helps prevent constipation by speeding up the passing of food and waste through your digestive tract.

Noticing the nutrients in whole grains

In addition to fiber, whole grains contain a variety of other nutrients:

✔ **B vitamins.** Like thiamin, riboflavin, and folic acid, the B vitamins have major roles in cell and energy metabolism, helping your body use food for fuel and create new cells.

✔ **Plant-based protein.** Grains contain varying amounts of protein that can help you meet your protein needs as you transition into a more plant-based Mediterranean diet.

✔ **Iron.** Iron is necessary for red blood cell production. Red blood cells transport and store oxygen throughout your body. Although vegetarian sources of iron aren't absorbed as readily as animal sources of iron, grains still have a decent amount of iron.

✔ **Magnesium.** This mineral is key for energy metabolism and a healthy immune system, and it helps you absorb calcium for healthy bones and teeth.

✔ **Phosphorus.** This mineral is needed for strong bones and teeth, as well as cell growth and maintenance.

Appreciating better taste

Whole grains, depending on the type, have a nuttier, more flavorful taste than refined grains. You may even find that white breads and pastas taste boring or bland after you begin to regularly include a variety of whole grains in your diet.

Understanding the Grain Stars of the Mediterranean

Say goodbye to low-carb diets. The Mediterranean diet is grounded in the practice of having a whole grain at every meal. And no, that doesn't mean eating an entire plate of whole wheat spaghetti with meat sauce for dinner.

Instead, people in the Mediterranean make their grains the side dish or create more of a balance by adding lean protein and vegetables to their pastas.

Grains don't give you only fiber and nutrients; they also add taste, texture, and flavor to every meal. The more variety, the better for both the nutrient value and your taste buds. In this section, you get familiar with the popular grains seen on any Mediterranean menu, the best ways to pair them, and why you should start including each and every one of them in your diet.

Barley

Barley is important to the world's food supply; it's the fourth most common cereal grain, after wheat, rice, and corn. But barley is consumed differently in America than it is in the Mediterranean: In America, much of the barley grown is refined down to create barley malt, which is a key ingredient for beer and is also used for animal feed.

Whole grain barley, on the other hand, is incorporated into Mediterranean cuisine. Barley is a real grain star because it has more fiber and more protein than your run-of-the mill grain. In fact, in ancient Rome, gladiators were also called *hordearii*, literally translated into "Barley Men," because they ate this grain during training to give them strength and endurance.

Even *pearled,* or *pearl,* barley, which is stripped of its outer bran layer, contains fiber and can help boost your energy and reduce your risk for disease. The reason is that barley, unlike other grains, contains fiber throughout its entire kernel, not just the outer layer. This fiber is largely in the form of soluble *beta-glucan* fiber, which has specific benefits to help reduce bad cholesterol and improve blood glucose levels.

Barley is not just for beef and barley soup! Use this nutty, chewy grain in any dish that would include rice, like pilaf. It's also commonly consumed as barley porridge, the same way oatmeal is made from oats. Or try tossing it into cold salads for a different texture.

Bulgur

There's no excuse for not including this quick and easy-to-eat grain into your diet. Bulgur is produced by boiling, cracking, and drying whole wheat kernels. The fact that it's cooked in the production process means easier prep for you when you buy it from the store. Bulgur has a mild flavor, and to prepare it, you just boil it for 10 minutes before eating.

Although bulgur looks like rice, it tastes more like pasta, so it's great for whole grain newbies. According to the Whole Grains Council, it's actually sometimes referred to as "Middle Eastern pasta" and is probably most commonly used in a traditional tabbouleh salad (a dish made with bulgur, tomatoes, cucumbers, parsley, mint, garlic, lemon, and drizzled with olive oil).

You can find bulgur in three grinds:

- ✓ Fine, which is perfect for tabbouleh and other salads
- ✓ Medium, often used in cereals like porridge
- ✓ Coarse or extra coarse, which is used for pilaf or stuffing

Nutritionally speaking, bulgur has more fiber than oats, corn, or buckwheat — about 4 grams for a half cup, cooked. So it makes a great side dish or base for a main dish because it fills you up on fewer calories.

Farro

Farro, also known as *emmer,* is an ancient strain of wheat that's making a big comeback; its especially popular in Italy. Farro is sold dried and is very similar to barley, but with a stronger, nutty flavor. When you shop for farro, look for the whole grain farro and not the pearled, or hulled, variety. Hulling faro removes a lot of its beneficial fiber and nutrients. Although whole grain faro takes longer to cook — about 50 to 60 minutes — it's worth the wait.

Farro is rich in complex carbohydrates and contains a particular type called *cyanogenic glucosides,* which has been found to boost immunity and keep blood glucose and cholesterol in check.

Use farro instead of rice in risotto, stir it into soups, cook it into cereal, or serve it as a side with fish or meat. You can also toss it into cold salads.

Polenta

When you think of comfort foods, your mind may wander to ice cream, potato chips, or something gooey and chocolate. In the Mediterranean, a whole grain — polenta — is a traditional comfort food! The word *polenta* is really the name for a dish that is made with a variety of grains, most notably cornmeal.

Polenta is very versatile and can be served creamy as a porridge, chilled and sliced into side dish cakes, used as a base for a sauce, or prepared with milk for a sweet dessert.

Because of the many ways that polenta can be prepared, it's healthfulness can also vary. Although originally prepared simply — just the grain and water — over time, cooks have added butter and cheese to make it more tasty. To reap the benefits of the fiber and nutrients like vitamin A, an antioxidant that helps boost your immunity and protect eye health, without toppling down the slippery slope of unhealthy fat and excessive calories, when using this whole grain, steer clear of add-ins that are high in saturated fat.

Here are some things to keep in mind when shopping for polenta:

- ✔ Look for the coarse ground variety or a package that is labeled "polenta." If the package says "degermed," it's no longer a whole grain.

- ✔ Polenta can be an excellent gluten-free grain option, but double-check that the one you choose isn't prepared with wheat flour.

Quinoa

Pronounced *KEEN-wah*, quinoa has come into the super food spotlight. Although not exactly technically a grain (it's a seed closely related to the beet family), it's consumed like a grain, so here we are. You find quinoa in the health food stores and in larger grocery chains. It's sold as white quinoa, red or black quinoa, quinoa flakes, or flour.

Although it's known as an "ancient grain" in the Mediterranean, it's really a hot new-*ish* product in the Western marketplace, for good reason:

- ✔ **High in protein.** Unlike most other grains, quinoa is a complete protein, meaning it contains all the essential amino acids, or building blocks of protein, that you need in your diet. It also has a higher ratio of protein in general, as well as fiber, both of which help to keep you fuller longer. By the way, quinoa also contains a small amount of heart-healthy fats to boot!

- ✔ **Vegetarian iron.** Quinoa offers a source of iron for vegetarians or vegans (or meat-eaters who don't get enough iron). One cup of quinoa gives you about 15 percent of your daily needs.

- ✔ **Gluten-free.** Because quinoa is gluten-free, it's a valuable food item for those in the celiac community, providing a dose of fiber and antioxidants, and adding variety to the gluten-free diet.

- ✔ **Easy to cook.** Quinoa grains can be cooked and ready to eat in just 15 minutes.

- ✔ **Delicious and versatile.** With a mild and nutty flavor, quinoa can be added to many different types of meals and dishes: added to salads, used as a crust for fish or chicken, made into gluten-free cookies or breads, stirred into soups . . . the possibilities are endless!

Rinse quinoa before cooking! It has a bitter coating that needs to be washed off; otherwise, it can impact the taste. For a complete introduction to this grain and over 100 recipes featuring quinoa, check out *Cooking with Quinoa For Dummies,* by Cheryl Forberg (John Wiley & Sons, Inc.).

Getting Practical: Ways Everyone Can Eat More Grains

Hearing all about the grains of the Mediterranean is one thing, but realistically incorporating them into your diet is another. You may feel like you need to be a *Top Chef* or plan days in advance to have one of these grains with a meal. Or you may be intimidated because you have a wheat or gluten allergy and know that many grains are off-limits.

For any lifestyle change to be effective, it's got to be practical for you. Otherwise, you'll do it for a week, maybe even a month if you're particularly determined, but then grow bored or tired with what you're eating and revert to your old habits. In this section, you find practical ways to enjoy grains, no matter what the situation. With the suggestions offered here, you'll be more likely to stick in the long run!

Swapping in grains at every meal

To make the transition into a whole grain lifestyle more easily, take it step by step. Table 11-1 gives you a game plan for adding in whole grains at every meal and tells you what you can ditch in favor of good nutrition.

Table 11-1	Swapping in Whole Grains	
When	**Swap Out**	**Swap In**
Breakfast	Refined cereals, bagels, muffins and pastries, waffles, pancakes	Whole wheat cereal, oatmeal, barley porridge, quinoa flour muffins, buckwheat pancakes
Lunch	White bread, noodle soup, croutons in salad	Whole wheat bread, broth-based barley soup, toasted whole grains in salad
Snack	Potato chips, pretzels	Air-popped popcorn, whole grain crackers
Dinner	White pasta, dinner rolls, white rice, breadcrumbs	Side of bulgur, polenta, farro, freekah, or even brown rice!

Taking allergies into consideration

Wheat and grains are often used interchangeably, but the truth is that not all grains contain wheat or gluten, which are common food sensitivities these days:

- **Wheat allergy:** People with wheat allergies have a sensitivity to certain proteins in wheat (albumin and globulin). Only about 35 percent of children who are born with a wheat allergy will continue with it throughout their teens, and it's actually very rare in adults. A true wheat allergy may cause indigestion, rash or itching, and hay fever symptoms.

- **Gluten sensitivity or allergy:** When people refer to a wheat sensitivity, they're often actually describing a gluten sensitivity or allergy. Celiac disease is an allergy to gluten, a protein found in wheat, barley, or rye that is often cross-contaminated into other grains like oats, rice, and corn. An estimated 3 million Americans have celiac disease, and many more have sensitivities to gluten and wheat.

Fortunately, gluten-free grains do exist! From the Mediterranean list, you can choose quinoa and polenta (corn). Other gluten-free whole grains include brown rice, buckwheat, millet, amaranth, and oats that haven't been contaminated with gluten.

Reading food labels is key if you have a gluten or wheat sensitivity. Any product that has wheat is required to list that ingredient on its food label. However, other gluten-containing foods, like barley, may not be required to do the same. Therefore, look for "gluten-free" on the label to be 100 percent sure.

Don't self-diagnose! If you or your child suffer from indigestion or more serious symptoms when it comes to wheat products, go to a physician for verification of what's going on. Unnecessarily excluding these foods from the diet can result in nutritional deficiencies. However, if you truly do have an allergy, you need to know so that you can be diligent with removing the sensitivity, becoming educated on how to make up for that nutrition, and preventing any additional health problems.

Cooking with Grains

After you've gone to the grocery store, picked up your whole grain, and got it in your kitchen, it's time to get cooking!

No rush on the storage front. Grains, especially ones with a hard outer shell like wheat or corn, can last in a cool, dry place for over 10 years. Grains that are "cracked" or hulled, or those with a softer outer shell, like quinoa or barley, can still last — not quite as long, but still for several years.

Depending on the type, the grain will cook differently. But in general when cooking grains, follow these steps:

1. **Rinse the grain before cooking.**

2. **Using a heavy saucepan with a tight-fitting lid, bring the water to a boil.**

   You need to use about 2 to 3 cups of water for 1 cup of grain.

3. **When the water is boiling, add the grain and reduce the heat. Then cover and simmer.**

   Use these times as a guide:

   - **For barley, farro, or rice:** 45 to 60 minutes

   - **For bulgur, quinoa, or oats:** About 20 minutes

   Reduce cooking times a bit if you want to keep that chewy texture of a grain. Often, this is preferred in traditional Mediterranean salads like tabbouleh.

4. **After the water is absorbed, use a fork to fluff up grains; then let them sit for about 10 to 15 minutes before eating.**

Chapter 12

Seafood and Animal Protein

• •

In This Chapter

▶ Fishing around for answers about seafood and its health benefits

▶ Incorporating seafood that's central to the Mediterranean diet

▶ Understanding how other animal proteins fit in

• •

Seafood is a mainstay of the Mediterranean diet and no wonder. The countries surrounded by the Mediterranean Sea have access to some of the most fresh and delicious seafood in the world! If you're a red meat fan, don't worry; you're still able to enjoy red meat in moderation. But the *scales* (pun intended!) tip toward seafood, poultry, and lean cuts of meat when you eat the Mediterranean way.

You may shy away from eating fish because you're concerned about contamination, and you've heard that toxins in fish can be harmful. Although these concerns are valid, when you make the right choices, the benefits outweigh any risks.

In this chapter, I give you the lowdown on the best fish to choose and delve into how other animal protein sources fit into the Mediterranean diet. One thing's for sure: You'll definitely see seafood in a different light after you discover the leading Mediterranean varieties and just how easy including fish in any meal can be.

Go Fish! The Lowdown on Types, Toxins, and Fish Oil Supplements

You may be a fish lover or a fish hater. If you're a lover, fantastic! You can eat a wide variety of fish, and this chapter may open your eyes to the possibilities. If you're a fish hater or have tried unsuccessfully once or twice to get into the fish habit, it's never too late to try again. Here, in short order, are a few key things to know about fish.

Recognizing the two general categories of fish

Fish are usually separated into two overarching categories:

- **Finfish:** Finfish are aquatic *vertebrae* (meaning they have backbones) animals with scales, gills, and fins.

- **Shellfish:** Shellfish are aquatic invertebrae (without backbones) animals with exoskeletons (a fancy word for shells). Shellfish actually don't technically fit into the definition of a fish, but they live in the water, and that's good enough for me!

Fish are also often categorized by where they are found (freshwater versus seawater) and whether they're wild or farmed. In addition, when you're talking about the best ways to cook fish, you can break down finfish by the color of the meat, their flavor, and texture. To find out more about cooking fish, head to the section "Cooking Up Seafood," later in this chapter.

Understanding the toxin issue

You may not fall into either category of loving or hating fish, but you may be skeptical about eating fish because of hearing about the danger of ingesting toxins when you eat fish. It's true: Some types of fish have higher levels of environmental toxins, such as mercury, that come from industrial pollution. Fish can absorb the mercury that's released into the water, and it builds up inside of them over time. Therefore, older fish and bigger fish who eat smaller fish, and fish that are farm-raised (versus wild) have higher toxin levels.

Women of child-bearing age, women who are pregnant, and children should follow this advice:

- Do not eat shark, swordfish, tilefish, and king mackerel, because they are high in mercury. Limit the amount of farmed fish you consume.

- Choose fish such as canned light tuna, wild salmon, shrimp, and catfish, which are often lower in mercury, and limit your consumption to no more than 12 ounces per week.

- Mix up the types of fish and shellfish you eat, and try not to eat the same kind more than once a week.

✔ If you eat fish caught from local rivers and streams, check advisories in your areas. If no advice is available, you can eat up to 6 ounces of this fish, but don't eat any other fish that week.

If you don't fall into those at-risk groups, you can be a little more flexible with the amount of fish you eat on a daily or weekly basis. Refer to the FDA's website (http://www.fda.gov) or the EPA's website (http://www.epa.gov) for more information about fish consumption guidelines and fish around where you live.

Remember, in many cases, the benefits of eating the fish described in this chapter outweigh the risks, especially if you're following the preceding guidelines.

Looking at supplements

If you've tried fish before and absolutely cannot stand the taste or the smell, or if you're allergic, you may try taking fish oil supplements to reap the benefits you've heard about.

Before taking a fish oil supplement, or any supplement for that matter, check with your primary care doctor or cardiologist. Fish oil acts as a blood thinner and, in high doses (more than 3 grams per day) taken with other prescribed blood thinners, can actually be detrimental to heart health.

Although fish oil is a popular supplement that gives you heart-healthy omega-3 fatty acids, pay attention to these issues regarding supplements:

✔ The FDA doesn't test quality prior to sale. Therefore, choose reputable brands with tested purity levels. I like the brand Nordic Naturals.

✔ Some fish oil supplements have been known to "come back up on you" — that is, cause a fishy-tasting burping, which defeats the purpose of taking supplements because you hate the taste. Choose a coated brand that's *enteric* (that is, broken down in the intestines). Doing so not only minimizes the burping issue, but also protects the omega-3s from being destroyed by your stomach acids before they're absorbed.

✔ In the past, research found that fish oil was beneficial for heart health and lowering triglycerides, but emerging research contradicts this claim when the oil is in the form of a supplement. However, the supplements may still offer the benefits of fish and fish oils described in the next section.

Seafood and cholesterol

Do you shy away from seafood because of concerns it'll raise your cholesterol levels? While seafood does contain cholesterol, you may be doing yourself a disservice by avoiding it altogether. Here's the lowdown on seafood and cholesterol levels:

✔ The American Heart Association recommends you keep your cholesterol intake to 300 mg per day or 200 mg if you have high cholesterol or heart disease.

✔ Seafood, particularly shellfish like shrimp and lobster, can contain up to about 100 mg for a 3-ounce serving. A typical restaurant serving usually contains much more than 3 ounces. Plus, being fried or served swimming in butter sauce tacks much more cholesterol (and saturated fat) onto your meal.

✔ Seafood is naturally low in fat, has virtually no saturated fat, and contains omega-3 fatty acids, which can be good for your heart. When steamed, broiled, or baked and eaten in moderation, seafood can and should absolutely be a part of your heart-healthy diet!

Seafood and the Mediterranean Diet

Conveniently close to the Mediterranean sea, it's no surprise that people in the Mediterranean eat mostly locally sourced seafood. Seafood, both fish and shellfish, are consumed several times per week. But how much should you eat?

Researchers out of the University of Florence in 2013 found that about 20 and 25 grams of fish (about 4 ounces) per day is the average consumed by the Mediterranean people. But you can reap benefits from including a 4-ounce serving just two or three days per week. Consider seafood a Mediterranean super food, as long as you choose wisely.

Underscoring the benefits of seafood

The main benefit of seafood comes from its omega-3 fatty acid content. Most Americans aren't getting enough of this essential fatty acid, and because your body doesn't make it itself, you need to eat it in your diet.

Eicosapentaenoic acid (EPA) and *docosahexaenoic acid* (DHA) are the two main types of omega-3 fatty acids found in fish like tuna and salmon. These fatty acids are easier for your body to use compared to the plant-based omega-3 fatty acid, *alpha-linolenic acid* (ALA). ALA is found in nuts, seeds, vegetable oils, green leafy vegetables, and fortified products and is converted by the body into EPA and DHA so that it can be used.

Omega-3 fatty acids' health benefits include the following:

- ✔ Reducing inflammation in the body, in the blood vessels, and in the joints, thereby reducing symptoms of arthritis, like stiffness and joint pain
- ✔ Lowering the risk for depression and possibly boosting the effects of antidepressants
- ✔ Improving visual and neurological development of infants in utero
- ✔ Possibly lowering triglycerides and reducing the risk for heart disease
- ✔ Possibly reducing your risk for Alzheimer's disease and dementia

The health benefits of seafood don't stop at omega-3 fatty acids. Seafood is a great source of protein and has all the necessary amino acids. In fact, more people globally rely on protein from the sea rather than protein from poultry, cattle, or sheep. You also get vitamins and minerals from seafood, such as vitamins A and C, magnesium, phosphorus, and selenium, to name a few.

Choosing the best seafood

Naturally, the fresher, the better when it comes to the quality and taste of seafood, but unless you're a fisherman or caught the fish yourself, determining how fresh it is can be a challenge. Table 12-1 outlines what to look for when you're buying fish at the store or supermarket.

Table 12-1	Choosing the Best Quality Seafood
Fish Part or Type	*Tips for the Choosing the Best Quality*
Eyes	Choose whole fish with clear and bright eyes to ensure you're getting the freshest possible fish.
Flesh	Flesh, like eye color, fades with age and becomes more dull. The flesh on fresh fish has a metallic and shiny hue.
Gills	When looking at whole fish, their gills should be bright red, not dark red.
Live fish	When purchasing lobster or crab or any other live seafood, the more movement, the better. Check with the owner of the fish market when the new shipments come in to ensure it's fresh.
Frozen fish	Although you can purchase frozen fish to retain freshness, especially if you live far from the sea, be aware that not all fish freezes well — oily fish, for example, doesn't freeze well. Great options for frozen fish include flash-frozen whole shrimp, octopus, squid, vacuum-packed scallops, tilapia, sole, and snapper.
Liquid in fish packaging	If the liquid is milky, pass on it. If you see liquid around the fish, it's okay; just make sure it's clear.

Selecting sustainable seafood

You may have heard the term *sustainable* in the context of sealife. The sustainable seafood movement started in the 1990s and has grown in popularity ever since. The term refers to catching or farming seafood in ways that protect the long-term health and well-being of different fish species and the oceans.

A variety of programs exist to raise consumer awareness, including the Monterey Bay Aquarium's Seafood Watch Program. If you go to its website (`http://www.monterey bayaquarium.org`), you can find seafood

that's certified sustainable. The site also lets you download an app that helps you choose the most ocean-friendly seafood.

A variety of certification programs exists, like one offered by the Marine Stewardship Council (`http://www.msc.org`), as well as chefs and restaurants who are more conscious of offering only sustainable seafood on their menus.

Here are some other tips to keep in mind when you're buying fish:

✔ A fish market should smell like fish, but it shouldn't smell like low tide. If it does, consider purchasing your fish elsewhere. Same goes for the fish itself. If it smells pungent, it's past its prime, and cooking or adding sauces won't do anything to solve that.

✔ If you don't have access to a fish market and live far away from the sea, avoid non-frozen shellfish. It won't be fresh, and you're better off with choosing frozen varieties or fish for quality meat.

✔ Smoked and canned fish travel well, but they may be higher in sodium. Nevertheless, they may be worth it because they stay fresh for a relatively long time, and they still provide the health benefits that fish offer. Here are my best bets for smoked or canned fish:

- Smoked salmon or whitefish

- Canned European tuna, sardines, or anchovies

- Water-packed tuna or salmon in cans or pouches

Meeting the Sealife Central to the Mediterranean Diet

Hundreds of fish are indigenous to the Mediterranean Sea. But this section highlights the top five seafood varieties that are typically included in a Mediterranean diet.

Salmon

Salmon is one of the top sources of omega-3 fatty acids, which is why it's at the top of the beneficial seafood list. It's also one of those fish that people who typically don't like fish will eat, and it can be prepared in many delicious ways: barbequed or blackened, made into salmon burgers or cakes, added to salad or included in spreads. (As you may realize by now, the Mediterranean diet isn't about deprivation, but about being satisfied with the foods you eat!)

Beyond omega-3s, a 4-ounce serving of salmon also contains your daily recommended vitamin D needs. Vitamin D is essential for calcium absorption to protect your bone health; it also helps regulate blood pressure. For even more nutritional punch and a crunchy taste, keep the omega-3 dense skin on, especially if you've selected a high-quality, low-contaminant piece of salmon (the toxins often concentrate in the skin).

Both wild and farmed salmon are relatively low in mercury. If farmed fish are fed more plant foods than fish, they have a lower omega-3 fatty acid content. Sometimes farmed salmon contain other toxins, like PCBs (polychlorinated biphenyls), but not all farmed salmon are created equal. When choosing salmon, opt for U.S., farm-raised Atlantic salmon or wild Alaskan or coho salmon.

Like all seafood, salmon can be fairly pricey, but that doesn't mean you have to do without if you're on a tight budget. Canned salmon is available any time of year, and it's less expensive than fresh without compromising on nutrition.

Sardines

Sardines are one of those foods you may scrunch your nose up at, even if you're a fish lover. But they're also one of the most nutritious foods you can eat. According to the USDA Nutrient Database, one 3.75-ounce can of sardines packed in oil contains

- 1.8 grams of omega-3 fatty acids. Although no an exact recommendation for daily amounts exists, this is probably within the range that most people need in order to reap the heart-health benefits.

- 351 milligrams of calcium (about 40 percent of daily needs). Don't scrunch your nose again, but sardines' thin bones provide much of this nondairy calcium and are good for your own bones and heart health.

- 8 micrograms of vitamin B12 (about 150 percent of daily needs), which is important for metabolism and normal functioning of your brain and nervous system.

- 365 milligrams of potassium, a mineral essential for proper heart functioning.

✔ 465 milligrams of sodium, which isn't great but at least you're getting nutritional bang, making them a much better option than overly processed foods with sodium.

Sardines are often canned, which preserves them (they're very perishable), but if you can find them fresh, they're even more nutritious.

Sardines are not only nutritious; they're also sustainable, devoid of toxins, and very inexpensive. To get the ball rolling on ways to incorporate sardines into your diet, try mashing them up onto whole wheat toast or crackers with mustard; add fresh, grilled sardines to a salad; or cook them with tomato sauce and veggies.

It's believed that the name "sardine" came from the Mediterranean island of Sardinia, where they were abundant. Now they're readily available in the Mediterranean Sea.

Tuna

Tuna is a popular fish in the Mediterranean and in America, too! Who hasn't had tuna salad or tuna casserole? Maybe you've even grilled a tuna steak for dinner occasionally or enjoyed tuna when you go out for sushi. It's a very versatile, delicious, and nutritious fish, full of omega-3 fatty acids, B vitamins, and *selenium,* a mineral that helps fight inflammation. Also, a 3-ounce serving of tuna provides 25 grams of protein, which could be about one-third to one-half of your needs for the entire day.

In America, classic tuna salad is often prepared with a glob of mayonnaise, adding unnecessary calories and fat to your dish. Instead, try the Mediterranean tuna salad (one of my favorite green salad toppers or sandwich stuffers): tuna mixed with olive oil, lemon, olives, onion, and often artichokes — no mayonnaise.

The problem with tuna is that it's high on the food chain and, therefore, one of the fish that contains high levels of mercury. For that reason, you need to monitor your consumption of tuna, especially if you are of child-bearing age or already pregnant. Canned white or albacore tuna is often higher in mercury than skipjack tuna (a tuna often used in Japanese cuisine); the FDA recommends pregnant women should have no more than 6 ounces of canned tuna per week. To reduce your exposure to mercury, choose a "light" tuna — preferably skipjack tuna. But remember, the FDA still puts a limit at 12 ounces of this type per week.

Mussels

Mussels are a type of clam. They have a lot of *muscle*, both literally and figuratively. The shell consists of two halves connected by a ligament, and internal muscles keep it tightly closed. To get to the meat inside, you either have to split open the shell using a special knife or cook the muscle until the shell opens.

Mussels, and other *bivalves*, like oysters, are environmentally friendly, improving water quality by feeding off the nutrients in the water.

You may underestimate the benefit of mussels because they're small or because you're familiar with them as *moules frites* (served with a plate of french fries). But a 3-ounce serving contains just 70 calories and offers omega-3s, vitamin B12, selenium, and folate, making them a valuable source of protein. So skip the fries, and eat mussels steamed or cooked in white wine, lemon, and herbs for a healthy and light dish.

Before being cooked, mussels (and all shellfish except shrimp) should be alive. In open air, a live mussel's shell will be tightly closed. If the shell is open, cracked, or smashed, assume it's unsafe to eat and discard it.

Oysters

Cultivated since ancient times, oysters are an important food source for people in coastal areas, and they are considered a delicacy worldwide. They've long been thought of as aphrodisiacs — possibly because they are loaded with zinc, a mineral that is linked to testosterone production (which increases desire in both men and women, by the way) and male fertility. Zinc is also important for your immune system and helps you fight infection.

Oysters last longer than most shellfish — up to four weeks out of water when refrigerated — and are typically served raw on the half-shell over ice with lemon juice, vinegar, and cocktail sauce; sometimes they're served with no condiments at all. They can also be cooked.

If you have a weak immune system or are at high risk for disease, don't eat raw oysters, because they may contain a bacteria that causes illness. Also, if you are pregnant, avoid all raw fish, which is more likely than cooked fish to contain parasites.

Cooking Up Seafood

After reading about the health benefits fish offer, you're probably ready to go beyond fried fish sticks or sandwiches and incorporate more varieties of fish, prepared in healthier ways, into your diet. Read on for key advice on how to prepare seafood for maximum nutrition and taste.

Like everything else you eat, cooking methods impact the healthfulness of your dish. So avoid fish that is deep-fried or overly processed, like fish sticks. Doing so helps you minimize the sodium and added preservatives you consume. Beyond that, any other preparation method is okay, as long as you don't add too much butter or salt to the dish.

For a fresh, healthy flavor, choose fresh herbs and spices (Chapter 17 lists a variety of seasonings to add), and brush on or cook the fish with extra-virgin olive oil. Fresh or thawed fish cooks quickly: it can be done within 10 minutes, depending on the cooking method (the flesh should be flaky and opaque). Here are some ideas:

- **Grilling:** Grilling cooks fish fast without drying it out. This cooking method is best with whole fish or thicker fillets, like tuna steak, salmon, or halibut. If you want to grill a thinner fillet, wrap the fish in tinfoil.

- **Steaming:** Steaming is one of the easiest ways to cook fish: You just place the fish in a stainless steel or bamboo steamer; you can even steam fish in the microwave. For a moist, flaky fish, steam between 5 and 10 minutes. Make sure you don't overcook it!

- **Baking:** Baking takes a bit longer than other methods (closer to 20 minutes), and leaner fish are at risk of drying out. To help keep the fish moist, add lemon juice or water to the pan, or wrap the fish in parchment paper.

- **Roasting:** Often used interchangeably with baking, roasting refers to cooking at a higher temperature in the oven (at least 300 degrees Fahrenheit and often much higher) to produce more browning on the surface and add more flavor.

- **Broiling:** Similar to grilling, broiling cooks fish quickly. For each inch of thickness, broil for 5 to 7 minutes. Also wrap fish in tinfoil to help seal in the flavor.

- **Poaching:** Poached fish is cooked in a simmering broth. This cooking method works for all types of fish and lets you infuse it with the flavor from the broth. If you're poaching a whole fish, wrap it in cheesecloth before placing it into the liquid.

✔ **Stir-frying:** In this method, you sear the fish in a wok (or a hot pan) with olive oil. For stir-frying, use a firm fish like cod or red snapper so that it doesn't fall apart. If you're stir-frying seafood like shrimp, keep the shell on so that it doesn't dry out.

Fitting Other Protein Sources into Your Diet

Fish isn't the only animal protein source on the Mediterranean diet, and it's a common misconception to think that no other meat is allowed. Poultry, red meat, and other animal sources like dairy and eggs certainly have a place in a Mediterranean diet.

The difference between the Mediterranean diet and a typical Western diet is that animal proteins are consumed less frequently and in smaller quantities. (Surprise, surprise — portion control is at it again!) In addition to keeping your serving sizes in check, you also need to know which types of these kinds of proteins are best for your health.

Choosing the best cuts of meat

Not only is meat a source of complete protein, containing all essential amino acids your body needs, but it can also be a good source of other vitamins and minerals, including B vitamins, iron, zinc, and magnesium. The downside is that many meats are also high in fat — the saturated, artery-clogging form of fat, which isn't good for your health.

The Mediterranean diet focuses on choosing leaner cuts of meat and having less than 3 ounces per day on average. Most of the lean cuts are poultry (primarily turkey or chicken), with a leaner cut of red meat eaten once per week or less frequently. According to the USDA, Americans, on the other hand, consume an average of 270 pounds of meat per year. That's equivalent to about 12 ounces per meat per person every day.

Finding the leanest cuts

To eat like people in the Mediterranean do, first you need to scale back your meat consumptions and incorporate more fish and plant-based protein. Then you need to focus on choosing the leanest cuts of meat. Here are tips to make the best choices you can at the grocery store or meat market:

- ✔ **Grade:** Refers to the amount of marbling in beef. The higher the grade, the more fat:
  - Prime is the fattiest.
  - Choice is moderate in fat.
  - Select is the leanest.
- ✔ **Cut:** This refers to the part of the animal the meat comes from.
  - Sirloin, tenderloin, round, or chuck are the leanest cuts of beef.
  - Loin chops, tenderloin, and leg are the leanest choices for pork or lamb.
  - Skinless chicken or turkey breast is your best bet when it comes to poultry.
  - Ground meat or poultry tend to use darker, fattier cuts and skin. Choose 90 percent or higher lean ground meat or poultry. After cooking ground meat, blot it with a paper towel or rinse it to remove even more fat.
  - Avoid processed meats like deli meats. Instead choose whole cuts to save on sodium and preservatives within.
- ✔ **Color:** In beef, you can visibly see *marbling* (streaks of white fat running through the cut), which indicates a higher fat content. White meat poultry is leaner than dark meat.

Trim off any visible fat from the meat or poultry before cooking. Doing so helps reduce the fat content even further. If you're roasting the meat, place it on a rack in a pan, which helps the fat drip away from the meat.

- ✔ **Grain- or grass-fed:** Grass-fed beef will always be labeled as such and is typically lower in fat and higher in omega-3 fatty acids. It will come at a premium cost but is worth it when it comes to flavor and nutrition. Also, bison, which is typically grass-fed, is gaining popularity. It tastes similar to beef but is lower in fat and calories.

Opting for healthy preparation methods

Just as with fish or anything else you cook, the good choices you make in the selection department can be undermined by how you prepare the food. Here are some ways you can incorporate meat into your diet in a healthy manner:

- ✔ Simmered in a stew or soup
- ✔ Baked for cutlets
- ✔ Ground into spiced meat patties or burgers that use spices rather than fat for flavor
- ✔ Slow-cooked with vegetables

 ✔ Grilled into kebabs and served over salads

 ✔ Roasted with potatoes

Be careful when you handle raw meat. Use separate cutting boards for meat and nonmeat foods, and wash any utensils and your hands thoroughly after handling. Also never thaw raw meat at room temperature. Instead, place it in the refrigerator to thaw. For classic Mediterranean recipes incorporating meat, refer to Chapter 16.

Meeting your calcium needs even as you limit your dairy

Although Americanized Mediterranean food may be rich in dairy, like chicken Parmesan dishes and Greek salads loaded with feta cheese, the traditional Mediterranean diet actually uses less dairy in general. Although you should eat dairy daily, limit your consumption to two servings per day of low-fat or fat-free sources. Full-fat dairy sources give you saturated fat, which isn't good for your heart. Nevertheless, whether full or low-fat, dairy is still a good source of protein, calcium, and vitamins.

Follow this guide to ensure you're getting enough (but not too much!) dairy in your diet. A serving of dairy equals

 ✔ **1.5 ounces of cheese.** In the Mediterranean, sheep and goat milk cheeses are more common than cow milk cheese, and they often contain less saturated fat. Common varieties include feta, Parmesan, ricotta, goat, fontina, and mozzarella.

When choosing cheese, go for unprocessed, natural cheese whenever possible. Also choose low-fat varieties (3 grams of fat or less per serving) or fat-free varieties (less than 0.5 grams per serving).

A "reduced-fat" label means that the cheese has 25 percent less fat than the full-fat cheese, but that doesn't mean it's necessarily low in fat.

 ✔ **1 cup of milk or yogurt.** Milk isn't consumed frequently in the Mediterranean, but yogurt sure is — and not just eaten as a breakfast or snack item; it's often used in cooking (tzatziki sauce, yogurt dips, and marinades for meat).

 • Greek yogurt, which has become popular in America, is made using a process that retains more protein and drains more of the natural carbohydrate (lactose) out. The result is a thicker yogurt that can help keep you satisfied longer!

 • Choose low-fat or fat-free yogurt (even Greek yogurt).

 • Avoid yogurts that include artificial flavoring or added sugar.

Dairy is a great source of calcium, which helps protect against osteoporosis and can help reduce your risk for high blood pressure. But it's not the only source of calcium in your diet. You can also get calcium from sources like these:

- Almonds
- Figs
- Green leafy vegetables
- Sesame seeds
- Salmon with bones

Factoring in eggs

Eggs on a heart-healthy diet?! Although they do contain cholesterol, people in the Mediterranean consume up to seven eggs per week, mostly in baking but also in omelets, soups, sauces, and desserts. The benefits of eggs, when consumed in moderation, outweigh any risk:

- Eggs are a good, inexpensive source of protein and are low in saturated fat. Instead, eggs have unsaturated, heart-healthy fat.

- They contain many vitamins, like vitamin A, folic acid, choline, and *biotin,* which is beneficial for your immune system and brain health.

- Eggs contain phytonutrients like lutein and zeaxanthin, which are important for eye health and slowing the effects of aging.

One egg yolk contains about 215 mg of cholesterol, but it's also the part that contains much of the egg's nutrition. It's okay to have an egg yolk per day as long as you keep other cholesterol sources in check. If a recipe calls for more than one egg, use one yolk and the rest in egg whites. Also, choose free-range or cage-free eggs, which have been shown to be higher in nutrients than conventional eggs.

Chapter 13

The Wonders of Wine

he Mediterranean diet is not a "diet" in the commonly accepted definition of the word; it's really a lifestyle. And nothing epitomizes that more
than the fact that wine has its place in the standard Mediterranean food
pyramid (refer to Chapter 1). It's true that wine can have health benefits, but
it also characterizes the Mediterranean way of life as one that values good
food, good drink, and relaxing meals.

Of course, drinking wine is optional, and (as you've probably noticed, if
you've read other chapters) over doing it with any one food does not a
healthy diet make. But drinking wine in moderation certainly fits into this
nutritious lifestyle!

In this chapter, you find out what "moderation" in the context of this diet
means and how to best pair your wine with food. In the process, you'll
become a bit of a wine connoisseur, knowing the varieties to buy at the store
and what to order when you eat out.

Not to be a buzzkill or anything, but in some situations — you're pregnant,
you have a health condition that prohibits alcohol consumption, and so on —
you should flat out not drink wine. And if you prefer not to drink alcohol, you
don't have to start just because you're adopting a Mediterranean-based diet.
Any health benefit that wine offers you can obtain from other nutrient-dense
foods.

Going Together: Diets and Wine

You probably don't see the words *wine* and *diet* going together hand in hand. But, as I say throughout this book, it's time to redefine your definition of the word *diet*. Think of it as the sum of what you eat in a day and not a restrictive, deprivation-type meal plan you may be used to.

Wine is a more natural part of the lifestyle and meal times in the Mediterranean than in America. Kids growing up in European countries are introduced to wine and beer in their teenage years and are taught that overdoing it isn't okay. Therefore, they're less likely to get drunk and more likely to learn and practice moderation, pairing a glass with a meal and then calling it a day. In fact, in countries where wine is part of the everyday living, alcohol is less likely to be abused, no matter what age the drinker.

Many people think that wine and alcohol in general may sabotage the ability to maintain a healthy weight. But again, in moderation, anything can fit. And when it comes to alcohol, wine is one of your best low-calorie options. Table 13-1 compares common alcoholic beverages and their calorie counts. (*Note:* These amounts are approximate and can vary, depending on brand and variety.)

Table 13-1	Alcohol Calorie Counts	
Drink	*Amount*	*Calories*
Wine	5 ounces	120
Beer	12 ounces	150
Classic gin martini	5 ounces	185
Margarita	5 ounces	350

If alcohol is a part of your daily routine, switch to wine to save calories and reap the health benefits outlined in this chapter.

If you take any medications or have any pre-existing health condition, check with your doctor to see whether alcohol is okay for you. Specifically,

- ✔ If you have high triglycerides (associated with heart disease and diabetes), alcohol may exacerbate or worsen your levels.
- ✔ If you're at risk for breast cancer, alcohol may increase tumor growth and estrogen production.

And of course, drinking too much of any type of alcohol lends calories without much nutrition, which can contribute to weight gain. Moderation is always the key. Head to the section "Raising a Glass in Moderation" later in this chapter to find out exactly what that means in terms of how much you can drink.

Factoring Wine into the Mediterranean Diet

Ever since the idea of a "French paradox" was observed in the early 1990s, wine and its significance to health have been the source of much research and debate.

The "French paradox" describes the phenomenon in which, despite a diet relatively high in saturated fat from cheeses, creamy sauces, and croissants, French people have a lower risk for heart disease. One original theory explaining this paradox is that the presence of red wine in the diet helps ward off heart disease. Since this idea was first proposed, a great deal of information has emerged on the health benefits of including a glass of wine every day. So drink up and read on to discover how a daily glass of wine can be good for you.

Red or white? Red, silly head!

The color of wine depends on the color of grape used. Red wine is made from purple or red grapes, and white is made from green or yellow grapes. Red grapes and wine have been fermenting with the skin on longer than white, giving them more antioxidants (antioxidants are concentrated in the grape's skin). One, called *resveratrol,* is especially important.

Research shows that all alcohol — red wine, white wine, beer, and spirits — may have health benefits, such as reducing risk for heart disease, heart attacks, stroke, and diabetes. In moderation, alcohol does the following:

✔ Raises your "good" (HDL) cholesterol, protecting your arteries

✔ Acts as a blood thinner, reducing formation of clots and risk for cardiac events

Red wine has the greatest amounts of antioxidants and has been more heavily researched relative to compounded benefits of the Mediterranean diet.

Red wines are classified by body type. In this context, *body type* doesn't refer to being pear-shaped or curvy. Instead it refers to the mouthfeel of the wine. Mouthfeel has a lot to do with *tannins,* a type of flavonoid found in wines (and which can also be found in teas). Typically, the more tannins, the higher the alcohol content and the greater the "dry pucker" taste you get when you take a sip. Tannins act as sort of a palate cleanser, too. Here are the different wine classifications:

✔ **Light-bodied:** Lowest in tannins. Examples include Pinot Noir and Zinfandel.

Rosé wine falls within the category of a light-bodied red wine, even though the color is a pinkish hue. Rosé is lighter than red wine because the skins of the grape have the shortest contact time with the juice. Rosés can also be made by blending together red and white wines.

✔ **Medium-bodied:** Moderate tannins. Examples include like Chianti, Shiraz, and Merlot.

✔ **Full-bodied:** Highest in tannins. Examples include Bordeaux and Cabernet Sauvignon.

Red wine has the potential to trigger migraines. The exact mechanism isn't clear, but research shows that tannins and *sulfites,* chemicals added to increase shelf life, may be two of the culprits. If you're susceptible to migraines, look for red wine without sulfites and avoid those highest in tannins.

Cheers! Looking at the benefits of red wine

Before you raise your glass, take a little time to find out about the antioxidants in red wine and understand how they impact your health. Savoring both the wine and its benefits is all part of the cultural experience.

Resveratrol is the magic ingredient in wine that has the greatest health perks. It's an antioxidant that helps fight free radicals in your body, boosting your immune system and warding off disease. Although it's unclear how much resveratrol you need (studies on resveratrol use rats and higher doses than that found in your glass of wine), resveratrol has been shown to have benefits in these arenas:

✔ **Heart disease:** Reduces inflammation, "bad" cholesterol, and risk for clots, and protects artery health.

✔ **Brain health:** Protects against cognitive decline and plaque formation in the brain, reduces inflammation, and may slow the progression of Alzheimer's and Parkinson's diseases.

- **Cancer:** Reduces tumor development.
- **Diabetes:** May help lower blood glucose levels and improve the body's response to insulin.

Wine isn't the only drink that provides your dose of resveratrol! It's also found in varying amounts in grapes, grape juice, blueberries, cranberries, peanuts, and dark chocolate.

Quercetin is another flavonoid compound in red wine. It helps widen blood vessels, minimize clots, and reduce inflammation. In addition to being found in wine, quercetin is also found in red apples, capers, dill, and berries.

Adding flavor with wine

Who says the only way to enjoy wine is to drink it? Wine can add a lot of flavor — without any of the fat — to many recipes. Using wine even lets you cut down on some of the oil you're using, which is an especially nifty benefit when you've already had your allotment for the day (refer to Chapter 8). In addition to adding flavor, wine also adds moisture. You can use it to make a mean marinade and to help tenderize meat. You can also use it as a substitute for oil when you're sautéing or simmering.

When you cook with wine, some of the alcohol evaporates away during the cooking process; how much varies, depending on the cooking method and length of cooking time.

When thinking about the type of wine to use in cooking, these guidelines may help:

- Choose lighter bodied wines for more delicately flavored dishes and full-bodied wines for dishes with more flavor.
- Use white wine for light colored dishes and sauces, red for darker-colored meals.
- Choose a wine you like to drink because the flavor will remain during the cooking process.
- Dry wine is low in sugar; sweeter wines have more natural sugars and therefore add more sweetness. When deciding which to use, choose the one that produce the flavor you're craving.

Choosing the Best Reds

Wow your friends with your newfound knowledge about the different red wines. To understand red wines, you really just need to know about grape varieties. Cabernet wines are made from cabernet grapes; merlot wine is made with merlot grapes; pinot noir is made from pinot noir grapes, and so on. Pretty simple, really (although it can get a bit more complicated for those grapes that go by different names).

Nevertheless, with this information, you'll no longer find yourself standing dumbfounded at the wine store or staring befuddled at a restaurant's wine list! Instead, you can choose your wine wisely and know what foods to pair it with.

Cabernet

Cabernet, or Cabernet Sauvignon, is probably one of the most recognizable wine varieties. These grapes grow pretty much everywhere that red grapes do! Cabernet Sauvignon is prominent in the French region of Bordeaux and is actually a blend between Cabernet Franc and Sauvignon Blanc grapes that occurred during the 1600s.

✔ **The taste:** Dry, medium- to full-bodied, with flavors like plum, blackberry, vanilla, and tobacco.

Cabernet and other red wines like Chianti and Pinot Noir are often fermented in oak barrels, adding a more robust and complex flavor to the wine.

✔ **What to pair it with:** Lean red meat, pastas, or a square of dark chocolate.

Chianti

Growing up, I remember my dad often ordering Chianti Classico to pair with an Italian dinner. Chianti is of the highest class, known as DOCG or *Denominazione di Origine Controllata e Garantita* (controlled designation of origin guaranteed), in the Italian wine classification system and is not only a type of grape but also a region where those grapes are grown in Tuscany.

✔ **The taste:** Dry, medium-bodied, with flavors of cherry and roses.

✔ **What to pair it with:** All Italian foods, tomato-based pasta, Parmesan cheese, and lean chicken or beef.

Merlot

If you're just getting into red wine, merlot may be the way to go. It's often blended into Cabernets to offer a softer flavor, and it has less tannins than the Cab, creating a nice balance between the two. Merlot origins can be traced back to France, and it's still a very popular wine in that country and around the world.

- ✔ **The taste:** Dry, medium-bodied, with flavors like plum, black cherry, spice, and chocolate.

- ✔ **What to pair it with:** Fairly versatile; enjoy it with poultry, lean red meats, pastas, and salad.

Pinot Noir

Pinot Noir is a tough grape to grow. It requires warm daytime temperatures with cooler evenings and a long growing season. Because of the strict conditions, you may pay a premium price for a bottle of Pinot Noir. But although this wine, which comes from the Burgundy region in France, may be fickle, it's worth the fight.

- ✔ **The taste:** Dry, light- to medium-bodied, with fruity flavors like cherry, blackberry, strawberry, and earthy tones, like cinnamon and clove.

- ✔ **What to pair it with:** Because it has a lighter body, Pinot Noir can work well with foods you'd typically pair white wine with. Therefore, Pinot Noir is one of the most versatile wines, going well with poultry, fish, and vegetables. It also offers a good balance to heavier dishes.

Lighter options: White Zinfandel

Also known as Rosé, White Zinfandel is made from red Zinfandel grapes, but the skins are removed soon after they're crushed, resulting in a pinkish or rose-colored wine instead of a deeper red.

- ✔ **The taste:** Sweet and light, with flavors like berry, citrus, and vanilla.

- ✔ **What to pair it with:** Because of its lighter body, like Pinot Noir, White Zinfandel pairs well with a wide variety of foods, from those that are mild to spicier dishes, fruit, fish, and lean meats.

Raising a Glass in Moderation

Although including alcohol and wine in your daily diet can have health benefits and increase enjoyment of a meal, it can also backfire if you overdo it. Raise a glass too much or too frequently and you'll be at risk for the following:

- ✔ Decreased absorption of vitamins and minerals from the food you eat, resulting in deficiencies
- ✔ Increased risk for liver disease
- ✔ Increased fat storage (your body metabolizes alcohol first and puts fats and sugar on the backburner)
- ✔ Lowered inhibitions, making you less likely to make smart decisions regarding food and a whole host of other things
- ✔ Weight gain (ounce per ounce, alcohol is more calorie-dense than most foods, except pure fat)

Liquid calories from beverages, especially alcohol, will not quench your hunger. Therefore, you can take in more calories than you may have bargained for before even starting your meal.

Knowing how much is enough

Everything in moderation! What does that mean when it comes to alcohol? One drink for women and two drinks for men, per day. That's it. And how large is one drink? Read on:

- ✔ Wine = 5 ounces
- ✔ Beer or wine coolers = 12 ounces
- ✔ Distilled spirits (80 proof) = 1.5 ounces

Be smart and stick to wine, light beer, or a spirit on the rocks. While a fruity sangria may be tempting, often the added sugar turns wine into a calorie bomb. In fact, any alcohol prepared with a drink mix, fruit juice, or soda can rack up the calories.

It's also completely normal in social situations to be tempted to go over the moderation limit, but remember, the people in the Mediterranean — or France — don't reap the benefits of wine from binge drinking. So to keep in check, try these tricks:

✔ Dilute your wine with sparkling water.

✔ Alternate a glass of wine with a nonalcoholic drink like water to keep calories down and prevent yourself from drinking too much.

✔ Don't drink on an empty stomach!

✔ Don't stand by the bar. Instead, get involved in the conversation. Socializing, after all, is what these events are all about!

When you shouldn't drink

If you don't drink, you certainly don't need to start simply for the health benefits. The beneficial nutrients like antioxidants in wine can also be found in foods. Plus too much of anything, especially alcohol, is not a good thing.

However, there are some instances in which you should absolutely not drink at all. When in doubt, you should always ask your physician or health care professional if it's safe for you specifically. If you fit into any of the following categories, forego drinking wine:

✔ If you're pregnant or trying to become pregnant.

✔ If you have a family history of alcoholism.

✔ If you're driving, planning to drive, or undertaking some other task involving heavy machinery or coordination.

✔ If you're younger than 21.

✔ If you have a medical condition that can be worsened by alcohol.

✔ If you're taking prescription drugs or other medications that can have a negative interaction with alcohol.

✔ If you're recovering from alcoholism or unable to drink in moderation. A hangover with a horrible headache the next morning is the least of your worries. Here are some sobering stats for you:

   • According to the Centers for Disease Control (CDC), 80,000 deaths in America every year are caused from excess drinking, making it the third leading lifestyle cause of death.

   • Heavy drinking can lead to brain damage, stomach ulcers, pancreatitis, liver disease, and fertility issues.

Part IV
Enjoying Life the Mediterranean Way

Five Ways to Create a Mediterranean-inspired Meal

- **Reapportion the food groups on your plate.** Divide your plate into quarters. Devote at least two of those quarters to vegetables and fruit, one to your protein source, and one to a whole grain.

- **Use a lean protein source and limit the amount to between 2 and 3 ounces.** Make seafood and poultry (lean chicken and turkey, for example) your main sources of animal protein and relegate red meat to a once-in-a-while treat.

- **Rely on healthy fats rather than unhealthy fats in your cooking and meal choices.** Healthy fats include olive oil, canola oil, avocados, nuts, and so on. These foods have monounsaturated and polyunsaturated omega-3 fatty acids — the kinds of fats associated with heart health — and less of the polyunsaturated and saturated fats that come from animals.

- **Enjoy a glass of red wine with your meal.** Red wine, in addition to enhancing the taste of foods you drink it with, has special nutrients, like resveratrol, that are shown to be heart-healthy. The key is moderation: one 5-ounce glass a day for women and two for men.

- **Take time to enjoy what you've prepared and the people with whom you share it.** The benefits of the Mediterranean diet aren't attributed solely to its dietary components but to the lifestyle components, too, specifically relaxation, family, laughter, and good times.

Being active is a key principle of the Mediterranean diet. Find a strategy that helps you walk 10,000 steps a day at www.dummies.com/extras/mediterraneandiet.

In this part . . .

✔ Choose a way to transition from your current diet to the Mediterranean diet so that you give yourself the greatest chance for success.

✔ Discover techniques that are integral to healthy cooking and learn how to prepare foods — like different kinds of whole grains or legumes — that you may be unfamiliar with.

✔ Save time and money when you're buying pricey or hard-to-find ingredients and devise tactics that let you reduce how long you're in the kitchen cooking.

✔ Prepare a variety of healthy and delicious recipes for every meal of the day.

Chapter 14

Integrating the Mediterranean Diet into Your Life

. . . .

In This Chapter

▶ Determining the best way to switch from your current diet to the Mediterranean diet

▶ Integrating a variety of spices into your dishes

▶ Discovering how to cook beans, lentils, and whole grains

▶ Adopting healthy ways to cook meat

. . . .

Weight-loss diets come and go, and most can help you lose the weight, but they aren't something you can live with long term. The focus of the Mediterranean diet is on your entire lifestyle. Paying attention to lifestyle changes, such as changing your portion sizes and exercising regularly, is the only way to see long-term results.

The Mediterranean diet helps you pay attention to the types of foods you eat, the portion sizes you consume, your physical activities, and your overall way of life. You can incorporate these changes into your daily life and create long-term habits that bring you *sustained* weight loss. But making a lifestyle change can be daunting, especially when that change involves food.

This chapter offers suggestions to help you successfully integrate the principles of the Mediterranean diet into your life. With the Mediterranean diet, you can still do all the things you enjoy, improve your health, *and* feel good about yourself, too.

Making the Switch to the Mediterranean Diet — Happily

Food is more than just fuel for your body. It's also the focal point of social engagements ("We're having a potluck at work"); the way a parent shows love ("I made your favorite!"); a treat to mark an achievement or milestone ("Let's go out to celebrate!"); an indication of health and well-being ("Are you eating enough?"); a way to commiserate ("She brought a casserole"), and more.

If you've grown up with a traditional Western diet, adopting the Mediterranean diet will be quite a change and will involve some key trade-offs:

You'll eat less of this	*And more of this*
Red meat	Lean meats and seafood
Saturated fats	Healthy fats
Processed foods	Whole foods
Refined grains	Whole grains

In addition, your serving sizes will change, as will the balance of food on your plate, with the protein and starch becoming sidekicks rather than the stars.

Of course, all these changes have very positive outcomes:

- ✔ Reduced risk of some very serious health conditions and diseases; Chapter 2 gives an overview and Part II focuses entirely on the health benefits of the Mediterranean diet.

- ✔ A introduction (or reintroduction) to how delicious — and filling — simply prepared, whole foods can be.

- ✔ An opportunity to maintain (or return) to a healthy body weight, without going to extraordinary lengths or having to do crazy things (grapefruit cleanse, anyone?).

So yes, switching to the Mediterranean diet will be a change, but it'll be a good one.

Still, change can be difficult, especially when it involves dietary habits. Not only do you have the logistical things to deal with (meal planning and preparation, stocking your pantry with key staples, fitting the supplies into your current budget, and so on), but you also have the emotional stuff: enjoying mealtimes, being happy with yourself, and, if you're a parent, feeling good about the example you're setting for your children.

So should you go cold turkey or take baby steps? Each has its advantages and disadvantages. The following sections describe and share the pros and cons of each. And because everyone's situation is different, we give you some things to think about as you determine which strategy is better for you.

Going cold turkey

Maybe you're someone who, after making a decision, embraces it completely and immediately. If so, making the switch from your current diet to the Mediterranean diet all at once may be right up your alley.

✔ **Advantages:** Hey, with all the studies pointing out the health benefits of this diet, who wouldn't benefit from making an immediate switch? Some health advantages — like lowered cholesterol — attributed to foods that are key components of the Mediterranean diet begin to show up in as little as two weeks!

✔ **Disadvantages:** Going cold turkey is hard. First, if your current diet relies on a lot of processed and convenience foods or contains very few of the dietary staples found in the Mediterranean diet, you face quite a learning curve (exactly how do you prepare an artichoke?) and a palate that needs to be retrained. Second, after the initial wave of enthusiasm wanes, you may easily return to your former diet.

Making gradual changes

In this approach, you make small, gradual changes. Maybe you adopt a certain cooking technique (using olive oil rather than shortening, for example), make it a regular part of your routine, and then make another small change. Maybe you start by preparing one Mediterranean-inspired meal a week and gradually increase that number over a period of time.

However you integrate the changes, the key is to do so in a way you can live with *and continue,* and then to build on that success over time. The method takes longer, but before you know it, your "regular diet" will be the Mediterranean diet.

✔ **Advantages:** Making gradual changes has a lot of benefits. Here are just a few:

• Even small changes make a big differences for your health.

• Changing one thing is easier than changing everything, and you're more likely to stick to a change that doesn't require a Herculean effort.

- You can absorb the cost of the more expensive staples (olive oil, nuts, and seafood, for example) more easily when you buy only one or two at a time.

- The children will be less likely to rebel and more likely to try something different when it's nestled in a plate of other things they know and like.

- You give yourself a learning curve that's more forgiving. If you discover that you really don't like chickpeas, you'll know before you create a week's worth of menus that include the legume in one form or another.

✔ **Disadvantages:** If you ask successful dieters how they find the willpower to choose an apple over a snickerdoodle, chances are the answer will be that they no longer keep snickerdoodles on hand. Your challenge will be committing to the small changes, even when other options are easily available.

Choosing an approach that's right for you

Which strategy is best? Whichever one works for you. Ask yourself these questions to find the approach that gives you the greatest chance for long-term success:

✔ **Do you have — and adhere to — a grocery budget?** A Mediterranean diet isn't necessarily more expensive than a traditional Western diet (see Chapter 15 for details), especially if you already budget for lean cuts of meat and fresh produce. But having to absorb the cost of a bunch of new and sometimes costly ingredients can be quite a hit if you have to stock up on the staples all at one time.

✔ **How busy is your schedule?** Let's face it. Cooking what you know — whatever that is — just takes less time than cooking something new, especially when that new dish also includes unfamiliar foods. If you have a hectic schedule, you may want to ramp up gradually rather than all at once. Eventually, you'll be whipping up Mediterranean-inspired meals just as easily and efficiently as you whip up a casserole or sloppy joes.

✔ **Is everyone in your household onboard?** Kids (or anyone else) who are used to chicken nuggets, fish sticks, macaroni and cheese, and mashed potatoes may need a little time to get used to the kinds of meals you'll serve on the Mediterranean diet. Yes, these foods are delicious, but they're also different. If your or your family's definition of good eats reads like a hit list of comfort foods, making small changes may be the better choice.

✔ **Are your kids picky eaters?** Which school of picky eater does your child belong to: the "I only eat certain things and won't try anything new" picky-eater school or the "I won't eat anything I don't recognize" school? Although some picky eaters may need an opportunity to get used to Mediterranean-inspired dishes (see the preceding item on this list), the diet's reliance on whole, simply prepared foods may appeal to picky eaters who don't want any surprises and don't like their foods touching.

✔ **Do you find big changes exciting or stressful?** Who needs more tension? No one. So go with the approach that helps you feel good about the changes you're making and doesn't add stress to your already busy life.

Still don't think you're ready to make wholesale changes yet? You can benefit from making smaller changes to your current diet to bring it more in line with the Mediterranean diet. Chapter 19 tells you how.

Boning Up on Cooking Techniques That Are Mediterranean Diet–Friendly

As discussions throughout this book point out, the Mediterranean diet relies primarily on fresh ingredients prepared simply. Nothing fancy. Nothing out of the ordinary. And no cooking classes required.

Phew!

It does, however, rely on some ingredients that you may not have had a lot of experience cooking (shellfish or whole grains like barley, for example) or other ingredients that you'll use so frequently that knowing the most efficient way to prepare them can save you time and hassle down the road. And the spices? If the salt-and-pepper seasoning regime is the only one you're familiar with, you'll find the kaleidoscope of spices used in Mediterranean cooking both beautiful and a little daunting.

In the following sections, we tell you how to cook, prepare, and creatively use many of the less-familiar items common to Mediterranean cooking.

A pinch of this and a pinch of that: Using herbs and spices

People in the Mediterranean use an abundance of fresh herbs and spices in their cooking. Besides providing taste, color, and aroma, herbs and spices also add health benefits to your meals.

Think about your own diet. Do you tend to use a lot of herbs and spices in your cooking, or do you mostly depend on salt and pepper? If you don't use many seasonings, your Mediterranean goal is to cook with more of them, both for the health benefits and to create amazing flavor in your food. This section lets you in on how to store the seasonings and how you can work more of them into your diet. To discover the health benefits of the key herbs and spices used in the Mediterranean diet, head to Chapter 17.

Storing fresh and bottled herbs

Herbs are delicate, so you want to make sure you store them properly to retain their best taste and their nutrient value.

Use these tips for storage:

- ✔ **Fresh herbs:** Immediately use them. Just like fruits and vegetables, the longer fresh herbs sit around, the more nutrients they lose. Store them in perforated bags in your refrigerator crisper for up to four days.

- ✔ **Dried herbs and spices:** Use them within a year of purchase. Keep them in airtight containers away from heat and light. You may want to record your date of purchase on the label; forgetting how long that stack of seasonings has been in your cupboard is really easy.

One way to ensure that herbs and seasonings don't sit too long on the shelf is to use them generously in your cooking. If you're running out of herbs every six months or so, you're on the right track! That's a good problem to have. For more information on the must-have herbs and spices in the Mediterranean diet, head to Chapter 17.

You may also consider keeping a garden for fresh herbs if you will be using them often. Fresh herbs are expensive at the grocery store, and they're relatively easy to grow, even in a city garden on your back porch. Check out *Herb Gardening For Dummies,* 2nd Edition, by Karan Davis Cutler, Kathleen Fisher, and Suzanne DeJohn (John Wiley & Sons, Inc.) for more on starting up your own herb garden.

Livening up food with herbs and spices

Figuring out a way to increase the herbs and spices in your diet, whether you currently use a moderate amount or none at all, is a great idea. Doing so adds lots of flavor on top of the health perks, so it really is a win-win situation. Here are some suggestions for getting more herbs and spices in your diet:

✔ Add ample amounts of herbs to your stews, soups, and chilis. Don't be shy.

✔ Use fresh basil leaves in sandwiches, or spread your bread with a basil pesto rather than with mayonnaise.

✔ Spice up a tuna- or chicken-salad sandwich with some curry, turmeric, and ginger.

✔ Let fresh mint, sliced cucumbers, and lemon sit in a pitcher of water for five to ten minutes for a refreshing drink.

✔ Mix fresh mint into your next fruit salad.

✔ Sprinkle fresh cilantro or basil over black beans and rice for a quick meal.

✔ Top off your scrambled eggs with your favorite herb combination.

✔ Kick up your lettuce-and-vegetable salads with cilantro and dill.

✔ Add fresh dill to fish.

Including whole grains

Although people on the Mediterranean coast frequently use pasta, they also consume many other grains, such as bulgur wheat, barley, and cornmeal. When you aren't used to eating these grains, you may not know how to cook them or add them creatively to your meals. Luckily, introducing them isn't difficult or time consuming. This section offers general cooking tips to conquer grain cookery, as well as suggestions for creating flavorful grain side dishes. Chapter 16 also includes some amazing recipes that feature whole grains to get you started.

Incorporating whole grains into your daily meal plans provides a great source of complex carbohydrates, fiber, vitamins, and minerals; it also adds flavor and texture to your meals. The trick is to use grains as a smaller side dish to avoid eating too many calories and increasing your blood sugar with too many carbohydrates. Use one-half to one cup of grains with your meals to stay on the healthy side of the fence. Refer to Chapter 11 for more information on the health benefits of whole grains.

Getting a handle on cooking times

Cooking grains is as simple as adding water and simmering. All grains pretty much cook the same way, other than varying cooking times. In fact, you can cook all grains the same way you cook rice. Table 14-1 lists cooking times for common whole grains. The amounts listed are for 1 cup of dry grain.

Table 14-1	Whole Grain Cooking Chart		
Type of Grain (1 Cup)	Amount of Liquid	Simmering Time after Boiling	Amount of Grain after Cooking
Brown rice	2½ cups	45–55 minutes	3 cups
Bulgur wheat — medium coarseness	2½ cups	None; remove from heat, cover, and let sit for 30 minutes and then drain any excess water	2½ cups
Cornmeal (polenta)	4 cups	25–30 minutes	2½ cups
Couscous	1 cup	None; remove from heat, cover, and let sit for 5–10 minutes	2 cups
Pearl barley	3 cups	45–60 minutes	3½ cups
Quinoa	2 cups	12–15 minutes	About 3 cups
Wild rice	3 cups	45–55 minutes	3 cups

You can batch cook a few pots of whole grains for the week to save time. Check out the Chapter 15 for more insight on batch cooking.

Adding flavor to grains

Incorporating grain side dishes in your menu can provide extra flavor to your meals. In fact, your grain side dishes end up tasting just as good as your main dish. In the Mediterranean region, people include a wide variety of grains in their meals; you aren't going to find a whole lot of plates with plain white rice.

Use the following tips to add some flavor and, in some cases, more nutrient value, to your grains (with the exception of cornmeal — its sweet flavor doesn't need any doctoring up):

- Add one to two teaspoons of heart-healthy olive oil or your favorite nut oil to your pot of grains for a light flavor. This idea works well if you have a very flavorful or saucy entree.
- Instead of cooking your grains in water, cook them in low-sodium chicken or vegetable broth for more flavor.
- Don't forget your fresh herbs! Try fresh basil, cilantro, or parsley.
- Throw in some dry spices such as cumin or cayenne pepper for a little kick.
- Sauté garlic, onions, and mushrooms and stir them together in your cooked grains. Take it an extra step and add some fresh herbs.

✔ Add chopped walnuts or slivered almonds to cooked grains for some crunch.

✔ Mix in chopped tomatoes and sliced olives for a savory flavor.

✔ Use 1 to 2 tablespoons of Parmesan, feta, or crumbled goat cheese in your pot of grains to add flavor and a creamy texture.

Don't be afraid to experiment in your kitchen. You may stumble upon something superb! To make a great basic starter dish that you can serve as-is or mixed with veggies, fresh herbs, and/or cheese and nuts, try this: Cook your grain. Sauté a shallot with 1 teaspoon of olive oil over medium-high heat. Add the shallot to your cooked grain with 1 teaspoon cumin, ½ teaspoon crushed coriander, ¼ teaspoon garlic powder, and salt to taste. After you get the hang of switching up your grain dishes, you'll never be faced with a boring side dish again!

Discovering beans and lentils

People in the Mediterranean often eat less meat, so they depend on plant-based protein foods like beans and lentils. In addition to acting as a protein source, beans and lentils are also packed with fiber, B vitamins, and phyto-chemicals (head to Chapter 9 for details). They're also economical and can create amazing flavor and texture in your meals.

Beans are available dried or canned. Canned beans are easy to use in any dish. Dried beans take longer to prepare, but they have better flavor and texture and less sodium than the canned variety. Lentils provide a unique, rich flavor and have the added benefit of quick preparation and cooking compared to dried beans. The following sections give you some tips on getting these Mediterranean staples ready to use.

If you aren't used to eating beans and lentils, gradually add them to your diet and drink lots of water to cut down on the constipation and gas associated with these foods.

Preparing canned beans

Canned beans provide a whole lot of convenience and still pack great flavor. You can pretty much open them and serve, but keep these notes in mind:

✔ If you're adding canned beans to a recipe, rinse them in a colander unless the recipe instructs you not to. Doing so removes the saucy liquid and helps decrease about 40 percent of the sodium used as a preservative.

✔ When incorporating canned beans into a hot dish that's cooking on a fairly high heat, add them toward the end of cooking. Otherwise, they can become too soggy and fall apart.

Preparing dried beans

Using dried beans requires a little bit more upfront work than using canned does, but your reward is a richer taste than what canned beans offer. Follow these steps:

1. **Sort through the beans, discarding any blemished or dirty ones.**

2. **Soak the beans.**

   Preparing dried beans for cooking involves soaking them in one of three ways:

   - **Soak them overnight (the most common approach).** Soak the beans in a large pot of water overnight (at least 8 hours). Afterward, simply discard the soaking liquid and cook with fresh water.

   - **Soak them in boiling water.** A quicker method is to bring the water to a boil, add the beans, remove the pan from the heat, and let the beans soak in the hot water for 3 to 4 hours. Discard the soaking liquid and then cook the beans in fresh water.

   - **Soak them in a pressure cooker.** For fast and furious soaking, use a pressure cooker. Add your beans and about 4 cups of water to the pressure cooker. Lock the lid on and turn the cooker to high pressure. After the cooker is heated to high, reduce the heat to maintain the pressure and cook for 2 minutes. Release the pressure cooker by running cold water over the lid and then drain the beans; they're now ready to use in your recipe.

3. **Cook the beans, according to the recipe or package instructions.**

   The upcoming section "Cooking times for dried legumes" offers general cooking information.

Preparing lentils

Lentils require no soaking before cooking. Just sort through them, discarding any that are discolored or have dirt on them. Give them a good rinse in a colander, and cook them according to package directions or recipe directions.

Cooking times for dried legumes

To cook unsoaked lentils or soaked dried beans, cover about 1 pound of the legumes with 6 cups of fresh water (not the water used for soaking). Simmer the beans or lentils until they're cooked and soft. Table 14-2 shows you some cooking times for various legumes.

Table 14-2	Cooking Times for Legumes	
Type of Legume	Cooking Time in a Saucepan	Cooking Time in a Pressure Cooker
Black beans	2–3 hours	15–20 minutes
Fava beans	1 hour	10–15 minutes
Chickpeas	2–3 hours	15–20 minutes
Kidney beans	2–3 hours	15–20 minutes
Lima beans	45 minutes	Not recommended
Pinto beans	2–3 hours	15–20 minutes
Lentils	30–45 minutes	Not recommended

Most people prefer that their beans have a pretty soft texture. If you aren't using a pressure cooker, you can try them at the early end of the cooking times to see if they're soft enough for you; if they aren't, continue cooking. Use your cooked beans within five days; if you can't make that happen, you can freeze them for up to six months.

Cooking meats the healthy way

Although the types of meats you eat on a regular basis are important, the way you cook them is equally important. If you deep-fry a lean chicken breast, it's not so lean anymore. So what do you do? Why, look to the Mediterranean, of course. Folks there tend to cook meats by using the following methods, which create a lot of flavor but still keep the meat lean. Table 14-3 lists the cooking options.

Table 14-3	Mediterranean Cooking Techniques for Meat	
Technique	Description	Good For
Braising	Simmering meats over low heat in a liquid (such as water, broth, wine, or fruit juice) in a covered pot for a long period of time	Chicken, beef, and pork dishes
Grilling	Cooking with direct heat over coals or another heat source such as gas	Any kind of meat

(continued)

Table 14-3 *(continued)*

Technique	Description	Good For
Poaching	Cooking meats gently in a small amount of liquid (such as broth or water) just below boiling	Meats that cook quickly, such as fish
Roasting	Cooking meats uncovered with dry heat in the oven	Large pieces of meat, such as a whole chicken, a pot roast, or pork tenderloins
Sautéing	Quickly cooking meats in a small amount of fat (such as butter or oil), stirring until the meat is cooked through	Bite-sized pieces of meat

More Than Food: Changing Your Life for Health and Happiness

The Mediterranean diet is about more than food. It's a way to embrace life to the fullest, to find peace and happiness in everyday events, and to stay active and engaged in meaningful ways. In fact, the benefits that accrue to those who follow the key principles of the diet itself aren't solely related to single foods but to the diet as a whole, which includes not only what you eat but how you live. The following sections offer suggestions to help you incorporate the tenets of the Mediterranean diet that deal with things beyond your plate.

Getting a good dose of daily activity

Historically, the people in the rural Mediterranean got plenty of daily activity through work, getting where they needed to go on foot, and having fun. Although you may rely heavily on your car and think such a lifestyle isn't realistic for you, you can still find ways to regularly incorporate activities that get your heart rate up and use your muscles. The following sections offer a few ideas. If you think of all the activities your life includes, you can undoubtedly come up with additional ways to embrace activity — without joining a gym.

Putting the car keys away for a healthy stroll

Getting in your car to run every errand isn't a way of life on the Mediterranean coast. Walking to the corner market or bakery is more common practice (much like a New Yorker's experience).

If you live within walking distance of shops or restaurants, give it a try. For example, if you want to go to a restaurant a few blocks away, walk to it and enjoy the activity as part of the experience. Or perhaps your child's school is within walking distance. Stroll to or from school each day with your child. You can enjoy each other's company and talk about the day as you teach your child the importance of taking a good walk each day. If you live in an area where forgoing your car for errands is impossible (such as a rural area or a city where walking isn't conducive), you can still look for ways to incorporate walking into your daily life.

No matter what type of city, town, burg, or hamlet you live in, try your best to take a stroll every day. Walking encompasses both aerobic and strength training and helps relieve stress. It can also help with weight management, bone health, heart health, and your mood and energy. Go to www.dummies.com/extras/mediterraneandiet to find a way to start walking 10,000 steps a day.

Finding fun ways to get daily exercise

Even though formalized exercise wasn't exactly a traditional part of life on the Mediterranean coast — we doubt that the old folks in Crete spent much time in a gym 50 years ago — you can incorporate scheduled exercise into your daily life to increase your level of physical activity.

Getting a little sunshine

The Mediterranean coast is so beautiful, who wouldn't want to enjoy time outside? Everybody's body needs sunshine so that it can produce healthy levels of vitamin D, which is associated with bone health, increased immune function, and lower cholesterol. As an added bonus, a warm, sunny day can go a long way to lift your spirits.

Note: Too much exposure to sunlight is associated with skin cancer and wrinkles. You can still enjoy sunshine in a healthy way. If you don't have personal history or family history of skin cancer, spending 15 to 20 minutes in the sun without sunscreen to produce some vitamin D is okay. If you're spending longer amounts of time in the sun, enjoy yourself with proper sunscreen and use hats and sunglasses for protection.

Make a list of all the physical activities you enjoy — pastimes such as gardening, swimming, hiking, jogging, bike riding, skateboarding, or skiing — and make more time to partake in those hobbies. If you love hitting the gym, by all means, add that to your list. Incorporating one fun activity each day goes a long way for your health.

Slowing down

If you spend your day going, going, going and fall into bed each night wondering where the day went or mentally ticking off items for tomorrow's to-do list, you definitely need to embrace the idea that slowing down is good for you.

If you don't believe that slowing down can really do that much for your health, consider this study: Researchers from the University of Rochester found that from Friday night until Sunday, study participants, even those with high income or exciting work lives, were in better moods, showed greater enjoyment in life, and had fewer aches and pains. And if just a couple of days of downtime can make a difference, think about the effects of making this type of time a priority throughout the week. Read on for ways to jump off the treadmill.

Taking time for the day's biggest meal

Even though the Mediterranean residents of days gone by were hard workers, often doing a significant amount of manual labor, they always made time for their largest meal of the day. Taking time for meal and family was a priority; you didn't see people eating in five minutes at the countertop.

Traditionally, this meal was lunch. Yet in many cultures, having a large, relaxing meal at lunchtime is difficult because of work schedules. However, you can adapt this strategy into your life by focusing on dinner. Prioritizing some time to unwind and relax from a busy work day provides other benefits for your family. According to a Columbia University survey, teenagers who eat with their families at least five days a week have better grades in school and are less prone to substance abuse.

Although taking time for a large, relaxing meal sounds like one of those optional strategies you can skip, keep in mind that even small lifestyle choices can make a very big impact on overall health. Family dinners can help you clear your head from work and provide enjoyment through good food and conversation. If you're go, go, go all day at work, prioritizing family meal time can be priceless for your daily stress management.

Making time for rest

Sleep is a basic, fundamental need that is now getting pushed aside by busy schedules. The average amount of sleep Americans get today is 2 hours less than it was 50 years ago. Sleep is crucial for proper health, and a lack of sleep can affect you in many ways, including decreasing your cognitive thinking ability (say good-bye to effective problem solving!) and increasing your risk of heart disease, high blood pressure, stroke, weight gain, and skin aging. For health purposes, doctors recommend you get eight hours of sleep each night. A Mediterranean lifestyle promotes rest time, including basic downtime and sleep. An afternoon siesta isn't all that uncommon.

Slow down and give your body the basic support it needs. To help you relax, turn off the television and computer screen because the light can turn on your body's "awake" signals. Spend some time relaxing before bed or curl up with a good book on the couch.

Taking some time to smell the roses

People on the Mediterranean coast enjoy all aspects of life including food, art, music, and nature. They fill their senses with great appreciation. When was the last time you listened to music or sat in a garden admiring the flowers? These small things can make a big impact on your health because taking in things that are beautiful to you is a significant part of relaxation and stress management.

Make time to enjoy these small moments. Go to your local museum, take a hike in the woods, sit on your front porch with a cup of tea, or go do some fishing along a brook. Taking some time to smell the roses may just be the best-kept health secret.

Working to live rather than living to work

In many areas, especially the Mediterranean region, working is a way to live life to the fullest rather than the main focus of life. Many people in the United States and Canada are working longer and longer days, and competition makes the daily grind feel like an unending battle to reach your career goals. Although the traditional workday is 8 hours, 10-to-12-hour days seem to have become the norm. If this description sounds all too familiar, work may be consuming more than its fair share of your life.

If you are working long hours and want to slow down, you can talk to your boss about a flexible schedule; perhaps you work a few longer days in order to have some shorter workdays. You can also set up clear boundaries about your time when you start a new job. You also want to work smarter and not harder, finding ways to decrease any wasted time during the workday so you can still get your work done, manage your competition, and have a life outside of work! Get tips for making a flexible schedule work for you at http://www.workoptions.com/about.htm.

Embracing life

No man or woman is an island. And one way to get the full benefit of Mediterranean lifestyle is to embrace the connections you have to your family and circle of friends and to allow yourself to discover and enjoy the things you're passionate about.

Enjoying time with friends and family

A hallmark of Mediterranean life is time spent with family and friends. In fact, many families in the Mediterranean have dinner parties once or twice a week rather than the once or twice a year as many Americans do. The fun and laughter that come with friendly get-togethers are vital for stress management. Without these little joyful experiences, stress can tip to an unhealthy balance.

Don't wait until the next birthday party or graduation. To put this strategy into practice, invite some of your close family and friends over each week, perhaps for dinner. It can be as casual as you like. Call up your family, friends, and neighbors and invite them over for grill night or the big football game. If you're new to an area, what better way to get to know people than to invite your neighbors for an open house? Find that sense of community wherever you live. The important thing is to add this type of fun and enjoyment to your life more often.

Creating a life where fun and passion are priorities

Enjoying life, having a good laugh, and making time for fun is a priority in certain regions of the Mediterranean coast. Fun is unique to you. Perhaps it means spending time with family, watching a funny movie, doing something active like skiing, or simply playing cards. No matter what you find fun, do more of it! Fun activities help you combat stress, not to mention make memories.

People who are passionate about and love life are happier, feel more fulfilled, and experience less stress. So what are you passionate about? Perhaps you love the arts, or maybe nature is your thing. Whatever your passions are, make sure to find a way to make them a part of your life.

Chapter 15

Eating Mediterranean When Money and Time Are Tight

In This Chapter
▶ Eating the Mediterranean way without blowing your budget
▶ Locating new or unfamiliar ingredients and foods
▶ Fitting time in a busy schedule for healthy cooking

*W*hen many people hear the words "eating healthy," they immediately think of two things: bland-tasting food and higher grocery bills. Add to that the claim that the Mediterranean diet includes dietary staples they may be unfamiliar with, and they may also think "impossible to find."

Well, rest easy. Those things don't apply to the Mediterranean diet. First, you won't find the people of the Mediterranean coast eating plain baked chicken and white rice. They're known for big flavors that utilize lots of impactful ingredients such as strong cheeses, fresh herbs and spices, vinegars, olives, garlic, and onions. Even quick, everyday meals are delicious and full of flavor. Cooking up some of the recipes in Chapter 16 can help take "boring" and "bland" out of your healthy food vocabulary.

When time and money are tight, adopting a new way of cooking and eating can be a real challenge. Yes, some of the ingredients are more expensive, and, at first blush anyway, preparing meals from scratch can seem more time-intensive than whipping up a meal from a box, especially when some ingredients are new or unfamiliar to you. But these challenges are pretty easy to overcome. Bottom line: To successfully fit the Mediterranean style of eating into your life, it needs to fit within your budget and your daily schedule. This chapter tells you how.

Staying within Your Budget at the Grocery

In most parts of the country, fresh seafood is a costlier alternative to hamburger, a staple of most family meals; leaner cuts of meat are typically more expensive than fattier ones; and fresh stuff — fresh cheeses, fresh produce, fresh herbs, and so on — is both more expensive and more perishable than the canned, frozen, and prepackaged counterparts.

Despite all this, the Mediterranean diet won't break the bank; in fact, the idea that it's expensive is a bit overblown. Yes, if the only change you were to make is to swap foods from one diet to the other, you'd suffer sticker shock. But if you embrace all the principles of the Mediterranean diet — eating smaller portion sizes, using unprocessed foods and whole grains, and taking time to savor your meals and your life — you may very well discover that you can eat just as economically on the Mediterranean diet as you can on your current diet and reap the benefits that come with being healthier.

Many of the foods that take starring roles in the Mediterranean diet are themselves economical. Beans, legumes, and grains, for example, are economical; add delicious plant-based protein, tons of vitamins and minerals, fiber, and phytochemicals (which help prevent chronic diseases); and are satisfying, which means you'll be less likely to snack on junk a couple of hours after eating a meal. Chickpeas (also known as garbanzo beans) and fava beans are two of the most common beans in Mediterranean cooking, but you also see other varieties, such as black beans and kidney beans.

Many of the vegetables and fruits of this plant-based diet — apples, broccoli, cabbage, grapes, green beans, lemons, onions, and tomatoes, for example, — are commonly available and affordable. Those that are more expensive, like olives, are available jarred or canned, which is generally less expensive, and pack so much flavor that a little bit goes a long way.

For the less economical ingredients or to make economical ingredients even more of a deal, try the strategies outlined in the next sections.

Buying frozen

They may not be as pretty (spinach brick, anyone?) or give you the same "I'm one with the land" feeling, but frozen and canned vegetables have just as many nutrients as their fresh-from-the-local-farmers'-market brethren, and they're often much less expensive. So stock up!

You're not neglecting your family if you serve canned carrots or frozen cauliflower rather than fresh. And although gourmands may insist that nothing beats a freshly prepared artichoke, who really has the time to work that little center piece out of the thing? Just pay attention to the role of the ingredient in the dish. If it's just a filler, canned is probably fine; if it's the main ingredient or is there to add crunch, opt for frozen.

Buying in season or on sale

If you're someone who creates a menu and then shops, flip those tasks: find what's on sale and then create your menu. If oranges or avocados are on sale, for example, add dishes that include these items on your menu that week. In-season items are generally less expensive out of season simply because of availability.

Local farmers' markets are a wonderful resource to get fresh, seasonal food for any community. Strolling outside through the aisles of the farmers' market helps get your creative juices flowing with what recipes you can make with these fresh foods (some which may have been picked that morning). If you've never been, take some time to explore your farmers' market and enjoy the sights, smells, and sounds. Check out www.localharvest.com for a map and listing of farmers' markets in your area.

Buying extra to save for later

This strategy helps save you money in a couple of ways: first, you're getting a good price now, and second, having the items on hand means you can wait for another sale before you have to buy again, ensuring you get a good price in the future, too.

Reserve this strategy for only those items that you'll use and are easy to store; you won't save anything by buying extra at a great price only to end up tossing it out.

Head to the upcoming section "Freezing for the future" for instructions on how to freeze many of the Mediterranean diet staples.

Buying from bulk bins

Bulk bins are great because the items are usually less expensive than the prepackaged counterparts, and you can buy just what you need. (No, you don't have to buy bag loads just because you're buying from bulk bins!) Consider buying these things from bulk bins:

- **Spices:** Very expensive when bought in jars in the baking aisle, spices bought from the bulk bins are often a fraction of the cost. The bonus? Buying only what you need is a way to ensure you use them before they go bad.

- **Grains and legumes:** Rice, barley, oatmeal, black beans, lentils. . . several whole grains and legumes are available in the bulk aisle. For the less-common varieties, expand your list of grocery stores to include ethnic food stores. You'll be amazed at the variety and pleased with the prices.

Freezing for the future

As we note earlier, a great way to save money and manage your grocery expenses is to buy extra when items are on sale and store them for future use. Freezing items is a great way to preserve their goodness and lengthen their life. Follow these suggestions when freezing several staples of the Mediterranean diet:

- **Meat and seafood:** Divide the meat or seafood into the serving sizes you'll use and wrap it tightly with freezer paper. The tighter the wrap, the better. Then label and date.

- **Nuts:** Simply place the nuts, shelled or unshelled, salted or unsalted, in a freezer bag, label and date, and toss in the freezer. Easy peasy. (The sidebar "Nuts to you!" shares how to store nuts without freezing.)

- **Herbs:** To freeze herbs, simply wash the herbs and allow them to dry. Then place them in a freezer bag and press out all the air.

- **Berries:** Wash and drain the fresh berries (you can skip this step for blueberries), arrange them in a single layer on a cookie sheet, and place them in the freezer until the individual berries are frozen. Then transfer them to in a sealable freezer bag, press out the air, and pop back into the freezer.

- **Cheeses:** Wrap the cheese tightly in freezer paper, label and date, and freeze. *Note:* Hard cheeses (cheddar, Swiss, and so on) take best to freezing, but you can freeze soft cheese as well. Be aware, however, that the texture will change from smooth to crumbly, so frozen cheeses are best used as ingredients in other dishes.

Here are a couple of pointers to ensure the safety of your frozen items and maintain their quality:

- **Make sure your freezer's temperature is 0 degrees or below.** This temperature helps retain the foods' nutrient content, color, and flavor. It also inactivates any microbes (bacteria, molds, and so on). In fact, food stored at this temperate is safe indefinitely, although the quality may degrade over extended periods of time.

✔ **When packaging food to be frozen, eliminate as much air exposure as you can.** Air is your enemy. It allows ice crystals to form and promotes freezer burn. Although these things don't make the frozen food unsafe, they do harm its flavor and texture.

Table 15-1 lists storage times for many foods. (*Note:* Because freezing at 0 degrees or lower keeps foods safe indefinitely, storage times are used to ensure quality only.)

Table 15-1	Storage Times to Ensure Quality
Food	*Recommended Storage Time*
Berries and Nuts	
Berries	10 months
Nuts	6–12 months
Meat and Poultry	
Meat, steaks and chops	4–12 months
Meat, ground	3–4 months
Poultry, whole or cut up	9–12 months
Fish and Seafood	
Fish, lean (cod, tilapia, flounder)	6 months
Fish, fatty (salmon, mackerel)	2–3 months
Shellfish (clams, scallops)	3–6 months
Shrimp	10 months
Cheeses	
Hard cheeses	6 months
Soft cheeses	6 months

Nuts to you!

Nuts are a common staple on the Mediterranean coast, used in salads, side dishes, and desserts. Nuts are a good source of healthy monounsaturated fats, but those fats can go rancid if you don't store your nuts properly. Use these guidelines for proper nut storage:

✔ Use airtight, plastic or glass containers.

✔ Avoid keeping nuts near high-odor foods such as garlic because nuts absorb the smell from their surroundings.

✔ Keep nuts at room temperature for up to three months or refrigerated for four months. You can also freeze them; refer to the section "Freezing for the future" for details.

Hassle-free Ways to Get Hard-to-Find Ingredients

One of the big differences between the North American lifestyle and that of the Mediterranean is where people shop for food. Many people in the Mediterranean, whether they live in large cities or small towns, depend more on local markets, butchers, bakers, and produce stands (though the big-box stores you're used to are popping up more and more in the Mediterranean). This dependence allows them to have fresher foods.

In most of the United States, taking a walk down the street to buy baked goods, produce, and fish from the local vendors just isn't a reality. So you have to make do in finding the right foods at your local chain or specialty stores.

Seeking the perfect seafood

Depending on where you live, you can find a good variety of both local fish and shipped-in fish at your local grocery store or fish market. Choose a variety of fish and shellfish each week. Your goal is to consume up to 12 ounces per week of lower-mercury seafood, including shrimp, salmon, pollock, and catfish.

Shopping local, no matter where you live

In North America, people often shop in big grocery stores whether they live in large cities or small towns. The conveniences of a big grocery store make life easy, but you often forego the benefit of seasonally fresh foods. Much of the produce found in grocery stores is shipped in from other states and even other countries. The longer the transport time, the more nutrients are lost.

Living in a big city does have some advantages if you want to shop someplace besides a large grocery store. A big city gives you opportunities to shop in specialty stores such as local bakeries and butchers. Take some time to explore your city and find these gems.

Although rural areas may not have the convenience of many different specialty markets, these regions do have their own positives for getting into the swing of Mediterranean cooking. For one, they may have more local produce stands where you can get fresh, locally grown fruits and vegetables. You may even have room to grow your own garden, which is the best way to get truly fresh produce.

If you don't have a lot of options or time and only can shop in your local grocery store, take some time to really explore your produce section. More and more grocery stores are carrying locally grown foods. It's usually not a very large section, but it's a great way to get some fresh, seasonal, local foods and still keep the convenience of your grocery shopping!

All seafood is good for you, but fatty fish found in cold waters such as the Pacific Ocean or cold freshwater lakes are higher in healthy omega-3 fatty acids. Leaner fish found in tropical waters may have lower levels of omega-3, but they're still a great source of lean protein.

You don't have to pick seafood unique to the Mediterranean region; rather, you want fish that's fresh, so local is better. And if you live near a coastal town, take the time to find a local market that sells the freshest catch. Nothing compares to fresh-caught fish for flavor.

Be aware that fish do contain mercury from pollutants in the water. For the average healthy adult, limiting your intake of the high-mercury fish listed here can keep you pretty safe. Pregnant women, nursing moms, women who may become pregnant, and small children should use the following tips for seafood safety from the Environmental Protection Agency:

- ✔ Avoid shark, swordfish, king mackerel (kingfish), and tilefish because they contain high levels of mercury.

- ✔ Choose light canned tuna as opposed to albacore canned tuna because the former has less mercury.

- ✔ Check your local advisories on any local fish caught in lakes and streams. If no advisories are available, eat up to 6 ounces per week of such local fish with no additional fish (of any kind) that week.

Chapter 12 has more details on the consumption guidelines and information and what to look for when selecting seafood.

Shopping for cheeses

Cheese is common in Mediterranean cooking, and you may be unfamiliar with some of the called-for cheeses (such as feta or goat cheese) or where to find them. Here are a few places to look when you're shopping:

- ✔ **Your local grocery story:** You can typically find containers of crumbled goat cheese and/or feta in the refrigerated section of your local grocery store or in the dedicated cheese counter. You can also ask your deli clerk if the cheese you're looking for is behind the counter. (The grocery's deli cold case is often full of unique cheeses, many of which you can sample.)

- ✔ **A local cheese shop:** You may be fortunate enough to have a store in your town that specializes in cheese. Count yourself lucky; you'll find everything you need there, plus knowledgeable clerks to answer questions and give you samples.

> ✔ **Online:** If you live in a very rural area and can't find these cheeses in your local grocery store, you can always shop online. Pricing varies depending on the stores. Here are a few to get you started: `http://www.amazon.com`, `http://www.cheesesupply.com`, and `http://www.igourmet.com`.

Exploring grains and breads

You notice a lot of pasta and rice in Mediterranean cooking, and you also see many grains you may not be used to cooking with, such as bulgur wheat, pearl barley, and cornmeal.

You should be able to find most grain products in the inner aisles of your grocery store, where you find the rice products. Cornmeal sometimes appears with the baking supplies. The grains that aren't as popular are often on the lower shelves, so be sure to look around. If you don't find the products you're looking for, venture to a gourmet grocer or health food store. You can also find many products at `http://www.amazon.com`.

Making Time in a Fast-Paced Lifestyle

A fast-paced lifestyle is part of reality today, but it also contradicts one of the premises of a Mediterranean lifestyle. When incorporating the Mediterranean diet into your own life, your first goal is to try to slow down. Look at all you have on your (figurative) plate and see whether you can start to say "no" to some things so you can free up time for yourself.

Prioritizing and putting together a plan

Overbooking yourself with work, kids, and other tasks is easy. Before you know it, you have no time for health and wellness. Children, family, certain occupations, and other obligations may make slowing down more difficult. However, you still can do a few things to make adopting the Mediterranean lifestyle easier. Keep these tips in mind:

> ✔ **Have a plan for your weekly grocery shopping and meal planning.** Doing so can save you time and help you to follow through with your food goals. See Chapter 1 for more details on how to make this idea work for you.

✔ **Pre-make meals and meal components to have at the ready.** Use batch cooking (see the later section "Making good use of batch cooking") to make meals ahead of time for later in the week or for freezing. Chop up a bunch of fresh veggies and prepare some simple grains like rice, quinoa, or barley at the beginning of the week to have on hand throughout the week so you can cut down your cooking time after your busy day.

✔ **Follow the great Mediterranean strategy of using fresh, raw produce with your meals.** Sometimes cooking all meal components takes up too much time. Add unadorned veggies such as sliced tomatoes and cucumbers or carrot sticks to your plate. Focus on easy-to-prepare meals for every day and use the more labor-intensive cooking for special occasions.

✔ **Embrace the convenience of the produce aisle.** Make use of pre-washed, pre-cut vegetables you can find at your local grocery store, such as salad mixes, baby carrots, grape tomatoes, and celery sticks.

✔ **Keep your kitchen well stocked.** That way, you always have Mediterranean foods such as olive oil and beans on hand for throwing together whatever meal strikes your fancy. Head to Chapter 1 for a list of foods commonly used in Mediterranean cuisine.

Scheduling time for cooking

Cooking is a crucial strategy in the Mediterranean lifestyle because it helps you lean more toward eating fresh, plant-based foods and away from depending on prepackaged meals or restaurant take-out. Cooking may already be a regular part of your world, or it may only happen once a week. Luckily, you don't have to cook every single day to benefit from the Mediterranean diet.

To incorporate cooking into your schedule, choose how often you cook on any given week. Managing your time and figuring out ahead of time how much you have available for cooking are key factors. Here are a few ideas:

✔ If you only have time a few nights a week, schedule those evenings for cooking and make enough leftovers for the next day. Treat this appointment like an important date you can't break.

✔ When you're planning, look at the prep and cooking times on each recipe to ensure you have enough time to follow through as well as time to eat. Too often people abandon the new, healthy changes they are making because of time-management problems. Here's what happens: You make a meal plan for the week (see Chapter 1), buy the groceries, and then continue on with your normal schedule. But then you find that recipe you were going to make on Wednesday needs 45 minutes of prep and cooking time, and you have only about 20 minutes to spare.

If you find yourself in that situation, feel free to make changes to your plans. Life happens to everyone, even the best chefs. If you get home too late one night to prepare your planned dish, postpone your cooking for another night and throw together a quick meal instead.

✔ Short on time every night? Choose recipes that take less than 20 minutes to prepare. For example, a small fillet of fish takes about 8 minutes to cook; pair that with a large salad and some crusty whole-grain bread and you've got a home-cooked dinner in no time.

✔ Utilize batch cooking. See the next section for details.

✔ Focus on one cooked dish rather than several for each meal. While your dish is cooking, you can gather fresh ingredients that require no cooking time (only prep time) for the rest of your meal. This strategy can help you avoid feeling overwhelmed in the kitchen. After you get the hang of it, you can slowly add another cooked dish and then another.

Living a Mediterranean lifestyle involves more time picking and preparing your foods than you may have experienced in the past. If so, strategize with small goals to help you start living this lifestyle. You don't have to cook three meals a day each and every day. If you look at your own habits, you likely cook part of the time, use quick pull-together meals like cereal or a sandwich other times, and eat out other meals. Whatever works for you is okay.

Making good use of batch cooking

Batch cooking is a great habit to get into, especially if you want to incorporate a Mediterranean-style diet but feel you don't have as much time to cook as you want. With *batch cooking,* you cook up larger amounts of food than you need for one meal and save the leftovers. The end result? A freezer well stocked with homemade items you can pull out for healthy, easy-to-serve meals later when time is short. You can more easily stick to your Mediterranean diet even when you're busy because you don't have to rely on prepackaged foods and eating out to save time.

Depending on your style, you can tackle batch cooking in a few ways:

✔ **Take a day to cook many items.** Get together three to five recipes, such as soups, stews, chilis, lasagnas, or casseroles. Clear off your calendar for the day and cook, cook, cook. Package your meals in freezer-friendly containers, date them, and place in the freezer for later use. Note that this strategy does take a lot of time and energy during your cooking day.

✔ **Spend a day prepping some of your go-to foods.** Instead of cooking several complete recipes at one time, you can get the base ingredients for later meals ready so you don't have to worry about them later. For example, you can precook beans, sauces, or whole grains such as rice or barley.

✔ **Make extra when cooking freezer-friendly meals.** You can then pack them, date them, and tuck them away in the freezer. For example, if you're grilling chicken, fill up that grill! Make more than you need and let it cool; slice the extras up and put them in individual storage containers. The next time you want to add grilled chicken to salads, burritos, sandwiches, or steamed veggies, you have the hardest part out of the way.

No matter what approach you use, make sure to package your meals in a way that works best for you. If you're single, use single-serving containers so that you don't have to warm up an entire dish. If you're cooking for a larger family, you can go ahead and freeze the complete meal. Keep a list on the outside of your freezer of the foods/meals you have stashed and dates you stored them. This way, you don't forget about the food you have (even if it gets hidden).

Chapter 16

Recipes to Tempt Your Tastebuds

. . . .

In This Chapter

▶ Exploring quick and easy Mediterranean-style breakfast ideas

▶ Using seasonal fruits and vegetables to create delicious side and entree salads

▶ Enjoying pasta without going overboard

▶ Preparing classic chicken and seafood entrees

▶ Creating amazing fruit-based desserts

. . . .

Bland, boring recipes are the one thing you won't find in Mediterranean cooking. The folks who live on the Mediterranean coast are known for big flavors in all their cooking, and the recipes in this chapter give you a glimpse.

Mediterranean cooking is all about exploring your senses through delicious foods. This chapter shows you how to make amazing breakfast dishes, enticing main dishes, and yummy desserts and snacks. These dishes prove how much flavor is possible with healthy cooking.

Waking Up to Breakfast, Mediterranean-Style

You may be surprised to hear that a typical Mediterranean breakfast is on the light side. Although people in the Mediterranean region don't skip breakfast outright, they typically rely on quick meals to get them through to the main meal, lunch.

A typical workday Mediterranean breakfast is often similar to a snack, usually consisting of two items you can throw together from your pantry. The most traditional Mediterranean breakfast options include the following, typically accompanied by milk, juice, or coffee:

- Toast with nut butter (like Nutella or peanut butter), fruit preserves, olive oil, or tomatoes
- Bread with cheese
- Yogurt
- Cereal
- A small pastry

Even though these items are small, they typically include protein and fat (through the nuts and dairy), which help you feel fuller and more satisfied until your next meal or snack. Small, easy breakfasts work well for anyone who has limited time in the morning — a characteristic that describes many people in the Westernized world.

Eating something small is far better than skipping breakfast all together, which may negatively affect your health. Research shows that beginning your day by eating a healthy breakfast is linked to

- Improved energy levels
- Weight control
- Better endurance for physical activities
- Improved concentration at work or in the classroom

Beginning your day with breakfast gives your body the energy it needs to get moving. Whether you're in a hurry and need to grab something on the run or have more time to prepare a home-cooked meal, the Mediterranean diet gives you ample options.

Similar to the United States and Canada, the weekends in the Mediterranean are often a time of cooking more elaborate breakfasts. To truly live the Mediterranean experience, choose simple breakfasts for most of your week and then enjoy a big breakfast a few days a week.

Mediterranean Toast

Prep time: 5 min • **Cook time:** 5 min • **Yield:** 4 servings

Ingredients	Directions
4 slices sprouted grain bread or whole wheat bread	**1** Toast the sprouted grain bread to desired brownness in a toaster.
8 tablespoons hummus	**2** Spread 2 tablespoons of hummus over each slice of toast. Top the hummus with ¼ cup sprouts and 1 boiled egg.
1 cup sprouts or micro-greens	
4 hard-boiled eggs, sliced	

Per serving: Calories 198 (From Fat 83); Fat 9g (Saturated 2g); Cholesterol 0mg; Sodium 288mg; Carbohydrate 17g (Dietary Fiber 4g); Protein 13g.

Bringing on the eggs

Eggs, eaten often in the Mediterranean, are a great breakfast choice because they're a wonderful source of protein and offer other healthy vitamins and minerals. Although they're high in cholesterol, eating eggs in moderation hasn't proven to have any adverse effects on heart health. In fact, a review of 224 studies carried out over the last 25 years has determined that eating eggs daily didn't raise cholesterol levels.

(Don't get too excited, though: Some other studies contradict this info.)

Doctors recommend a 300-milligrams-of-cholesterol per day limit (one large egg has 213 milligrams of cholesterol, all in the yolk) for the average healthy person. If you have high cholesterol or heart disease, be sure to follow your own physician's specific recommendations.

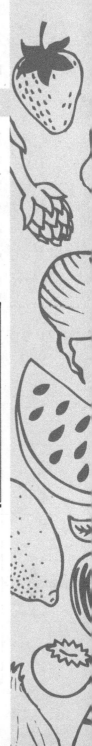

Overnight Muesli

Prep time: 5 min • **Yield:** 4 servings

Ingredients	*Directions*
1½ cups old fashioned oats 1 cup puffed rice cereal ¼ cup dried apricots, chopped ¼ cup sunflower seeds	**1** In a large mixing bowl, mix together the oats, rice cereal, apricots, sunflower seeds, walnuts, and raisins. Sprinkle the cardamom (or cinnamon) over the top and stir well.
¼ cup walnuts ¼ cup raisins ½ teaspoon ground cardamom or cinnamon	**2** Divide the muesli among four bowls (each bowl will have approximately a heaping ¾ cup of the mixture). Top each serving of muesli with 1 tablespoon honey, 1 cup of milk, and then stir well. Cover and refrigerate the mixture over night.
4 tablespoons honey 4 cups low-fat milk	**3** In the morning, simply stir and then serve.

Per serving: Calories 437 (From Fat 118); Fat 13g (Saturated 3g); Cholesterol 12mg; Sodium 113mg; Carbohydrate 69g (Dietary Fiber 6g); Protein 16g.

A spoonful of honey makes the cold symptoms go away

Honey is a popular ingredient in Mediterranean cooking and also has some interesting health benefits along with its sweet, satisfying flavor. In a small study, researchers from Penn State College of Medicine found that a single nighttime dose of buckwheat honey helped to alleviate cough in kids age 2 to 18 with upper respiratory tract infections. A spoonful of honey beats cough medicine any day!

Another study from the University of Ottawa found that two specific types of honey —

manuka and sidr — were effective at killing off bacteria associated with sinusitis. Chronic sinusitis occurs when the nasal membranes become inflamed, leading to stuffy nose, headaches, and difficulty breathing.

More research is needed in this area, but the good news is that a little honey is certainly not bad for you. If you're battling a cold or have sinusitis, give honey a try.

Spinach and Sausage Breakfast Casserole

Prep time: 20 min • **Cook time:** 30 min • **Yield:** 10 servings

Ingredients	Directions
1 pound bulk chicken or turkey breast sausage	**1** Preheat the oven to 400 degrees. Grease a 9-x-13-inch baking dish and set aside.
¼ cup chopped scallions	
2 cloves garlic, peeled and minced	**2** Cook the sausage over medium heat in a large skillet, breaking it up as it cooks. Add the scallions and cook until the meat is no longer pink. Add the garlic and cook for 1 minute, or until the garlic is fragrant. Drain any fat from the pan.
1 package (10 ounces) frozen chopped spinach, thawed and squeezed dry	
8 ounces mozzarella cheese, shredded	**3** Add the spinach to the skillet with the sausage and mix together until the ingredients are thoroughly combined. Transfer the sausage-spinach mixture to the prepared baking dish and sprinkle the mixture with the mozzarella cheese.
1½ cups nonfat Greek yogurt	
3 eggs	
8 slices of whole wheat bread, cut into 1-inch cubes	**4** In a small bowl, whisk together the yogurt and eggs; fold in the bread cubes. Pour the egg-bread mixture evenly over the sausage mixture. Gently rap the dish against the counter once or twice to make sure the liquid is evenly distributed.
2 tablespoons grated Parmesan cheese	
	5 Bake for 30 minutes, or until a thermometer inserted in the center reads 160 degrees. Sprinkle the casserole with the Parmesan cheese and bake for 5 more minutes, or until bubbly. Let the dish sit for 10 minutes before serving.

Per serving: Calories 243 (From Fat 100); Fat 11g (Saturated 5g); Cholesterol 106mg; Sodium 565mg; Carbohydrate 13g (Dietary Fiber 2g); Protein 22g.

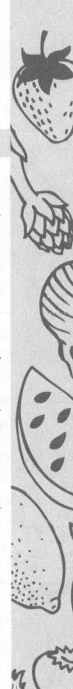

Avocado Smoothie

Prep time: 5 min • **Yield:** 4 servings

Ingredients	Directions
1 avocado, peeled and pitted	*1* Place all of the ingredients into a blender and blend on high until smooth.
2 bananas, frozen	
1 cup honey Greek yogurt	
2 cups low-fat milk	

Per serving: Calories 241 (From Fat 77); Fat 9g (Saturated 3g); Cholesterol 8mg; Sodium 69mg; Carbohydrate 24g (Dietary Fiber 5g); Protein 10g.

Tip: To make this smoothie colder or thicker, you can add some ice cubes to the blender with the other ingredients.

Vary It! Craving chocolate? Add in 1 tablespoon cocoa powder! It's packed with antioxidants and fiber and satisfies sweet cravings.

Fact about avocados

Avocados are one of the healthiest foods you can eat. Creamy, delicately flavored, and good alone, as part of dips or spreads, or sliced on sandwiches, avocados are also a good source of nutrients. A whole, medium-sized (5-ounce) avocado has about 250 calories and is a good source of protein, potassium, healthy fats, dietary fiber, folate, vitamin A, magnesium, and more.

To get the flesh out of an avocado, follow these easy steps:

1. With a sharp knife, carefully cut through the skin and flesh until the blade hits the seed and then, keeping the knife in position, cut around the seed without lifting the knife from the flesh.

2. Holding one half of the scored avocado in the palm of one hand, twist and lift the other half off the seed.

3. With the bottom half still in your palm, carefully hit the seed with the knife blade, hard enough to penetrate the seed about a quarter-inch deep; without removing the knife, twist and lift the seed free.

4. Use a large spoon to scoop the flesh from the skin.

You can now slice or otherwise prepare the avocado as you like. Store whatever you don't use in a plastic bag in the refrigerator.

Note: The flesh will darken very quickly once exposed to air. To keep it from doing so, sprinkle it with lemon juice. If you plan to use only half of the avocado, leave the unused half in its skin to minimize the amount of exposed flesh and store as usual.

Lighter Fare: Soup, Salad, and Sandwiches

Whether you're preparing a lunch or light dinner, soups, salads and sandwiches are the go-to items. They are also good options when served as part of a larger meal.

Use the recipes in this section as they are or feel free to celebrate the way the people of the Mediterranean live by substituting vegetables and herbs according to your taste and what you have on hand.

Warming up with a great cup of soup

No one does soup better than the people who live on the coast of the Mediterranean. Not only do soups and stews incorporate flavors and ingredients unique to the region, but they also have many health benefits, including the following:

- Soups and stews that include vegetables, beans, and/or lentils are full of fiber, which helps with weight management (because it helps you feel full on fewer calories), lowers bad cholesterol, and manages blood sugar levels.

- Hot soups cause you to eat more slowly, which gives your brain time to feel more satisfied with fewer calories.

- The variety of vegetables, herbs, lentils, and beans in many soups gives you a big dose of vitamins, minerals, and phytonutrients for disease prevention and general wellness.

Soups can be used as a starter or as the entire meal in itself and are a great way to add a variety of nutrients to your diet.

Going green and leafy: Salads

In the Mediterranean, salads are often the starter for a meal, but you can also find some regions that eat the salad after the main course. Bean salads and other vegetable salads make a popular side with a meal, and some salads are big enough to be the entire meal. Health-wise, all these options are great ways to get those extra veggies!

Making salads a regular part of your dining experience is a good habit to get into for several reasons:

- They help you feel full even though you're taking in fewer calories (depending on the toppings and amount of dressing).

- They increase your intake of vitamins, minerals, and phytochemicals, helping you to prevent diseases.

- They add more fiber in your diet, which helps with weight management, colon health, and heart health.

Picking the best greens for your next salad

Not too long ago, the main selections of salad greens you'd find in your local grocery store pretty much began and ended with iceberg, romaine, and red leaf lettuces. Now you can find a whole assortment of greens you can purchase separately or prewashed and mixed together in bags. Knowing what flavors to expect can help you pick the right greens for your salads. Use these descriptions to help you navigate the world of salad greens:

- **Iceberg lettuce:** Pale, crisp iceberg lettuce has a mild flavor due to its high water content. This salad green is great to add to other salad mixes for a crunchy texture. Although iceberg isn't nutrient-dense, it's low in calories and helps improve your water intake.

- **Romaine lettuce:** Romaine is a large leaf with a white stem that provides a crunchier texture to your salad. The flavor is mild and can be a wonderful addition to any salad combination.

- **Leaf lettuce:** Green leaf and red leaf lettuce are popular in American cuisine. They have a light flavor, and their uneven leaves provide lots of great texture for any salad base.

- **Arugula:** Arugula originates from the Mediterranean coast and has a bitter, peppery flavor you won't mistake for any other green. If you're looking for strong flavor to add a special kick, arugula's your leaf.

- **Butterhead:** Butterhead, or bibb, lettuce has a very soft, delicate texture and a full flavor. This lettuce is a little on the pricey side, so you can also use its sister lettuce, Boston butterhead, which isn't as soft but is similar in texture and taste. You can use these lettuces as a base in any salad; they go very nicely with fruit.

- **Dandelion greens:** Dandelion greens have a bitter flavor and delicate texture, adding a big punch of flavor to your next mixed green salad. To balance out the strong flavor, combine these greens with milder flavors such as green leaf or romaine. Dandelion greens also go well with salty flavors such as olives or capers.

Mixing up salad dressings the Mediterranean way

One thing you won't find in the traditional Mediterranean refrigerator is several bottles of salad dressings such as ranch, Thousand Island, or even Italian. Instead, people in that region make their own dressings out of basic ingredients each time they prepare a salad. Although this practice may seem like too much work to you, it's really simple — honest. Most Mediterranean salad dressings include the following:

- A high-quality extra-virgin olive oil
- Vinegar (red wine, balsamic, or other infused or flavored vinegars)
- Salt

That about sums it up. The flavors and acidity level of your vinegar will dictate how much you use, but start with your olive oil, add a little vinegar and a pinch of salt, whisk it together in a small bowl or shake it in a bottle, and see how it tastes by dipping a leaf of lettuce. Although you can find some specific recipes on the Internet, you'll probably do best by playing around with this basic recipe, in true Mediterranean fashion, until you perfect it to your specific taste. If you're feeling really crazy, you can try adding lemon juice, garlic, or a dash of mustard. Before you know it, you'll have your own perfected signature salad dressing.

Add fresh herbs and strong flavors such as sliced onions directly to your salads instead of adding these elements to your dressing.

Making sensational sandwiches

Different styles of sandwiches are popular in many countries, especially on the Mediterranean coast, as a quick, casual food. Pairing bread with a variety of meats, cheeses, and vegetables makes using foods you have on hand (and cleaning up those leftovers) easy.

Italians in particular love bread, and you see it used in many different ways throughout their cooking. *Paninis* are a popular style of Italian sandwich that involves smashing the final sandwich between hot irons similar to a waffle iron. Of course, big crusty bread topped with local favorites like vegetables and seafood is another common choice. So throw out those boring old peanut butter and jelly sandwiches and try this section's Mediterranean-inspired dish.

Here are some tips to make a boring sandwich sensational while keeping it sensible:

- ✔ **Begin with the right breads:** Some breads are healthier than others. Choose whole-grain breads, sourdough bread, and whole-wheat pitas for more fiber for digestive and heart health. Fiber also helps you feel fuller longer.

- ✔ **Choose lean cuts of meat:** Go for lean meats like turkey or chicken breast; if you can't resist the higher-calorie and -fat meats like beef, layer them lightly.

- ✔ **Opt for stronger-flavored cheeses:** Use a small amount of a strong-flavored cheese such as feta or goat cheese to maximize taste without going overboard on fat and calories. And go easy on melting layers of cheese on your sandwiches; add tomatoes and basil leaves instead.

- ✔ **Add vegetables:** Piling on simple vegetables such as dark leafy greens, tomatoes, and cucumbers can pack plenty of flavor and nutrients. Try adding cooked veggies to your sandwich as well.

- ✔ **Include fresh herbs:** Fresh herbs like basil leaves can add big flavor to your next sandwich, and they contain important nutrients and phytochemicals to help you stay healthy and combat diseases. Use fresh dill with fish sandwiches or sprinkle a little fresh cilantro on a turkey sandwich.

- ✔ **Balance light with heavy:** Combine heavy foods with light foods for better balance. If you're eating a beef sandwich at a restaurant, opt for a salad or soup rather than the French fries or potato chips or get just half a sandwich.

- ✔ **Choose healthier spreads and condiments:** Try some healthier and tastier spreads: Brush olive oil on your bread in place of butter when making a hot sandwich. Spread hummus, pesto, or avocado on a cold sandwich. These swaps add more nutrients and help you switch to healthy fats.

TIP

A soup-er weight-loss tip

Enjoying a cup of soup before your meal may just help you lose weight, according to researchers at Pennsylvania State University. They found that participants who ate a low-calorie vegetable/broth-based soup prior to a meal ate one-fifth fewer calories for the total meal than those who ate the entree alone.

This finding makes sense because as you begin to eat, hormones begin telling your brain you are full. Of course, this strategy only works if you eat a low-calorie soup; otherwise, the calories add up, and you don't really reduce the calorie count of your meal.

Avocado and Strawberry Salad with Sweet Balsamic Dressing

Prep time: 15 min • **Yield:** 4 servings

Ingredients	*Directions*
8 cups baby arugula or baby spinach 1 large avocado, peeled and diced 12 strawberries, hulled and sliced ¼ cup pumpkin or sunflower seeds ¼ cup feta cheese, crumbled ½ cup balsamic vinegar 2 tablespoons honey ¼ cup olive oil	**1** Place the baby greens on a large serving platter. Top the greems with the avocado, strawberry slices, pumpkin seeds, and feta cheese. Cover and chill the salad in the refrigerator until ready to serve. **2** Meanwhile, in a small saucepan heat the balsamic vinegar and honey over medium-high heat for 5 minutes. Whisk the olive oil into the vinegar until well blended and then drizzle the dressing over the salad. Serve.

Per serving: Calories 367 (From Fat 244); Fat 27g (Saturated 6g); Cholesterol 8mg; Sodium 126mg; Carbohydrate 27g (Dietary Fiber 7g); Protein 7g.

Tip: Coping with high cholesterol? Top this salad with orange zest, which is currently being researched for its cholesterol-lowering properties!

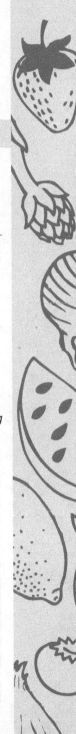

Spiced Chickpea Soup

Prep time: 10 min • **Cook time:** 20 min • **Yield:** 4 servings

Ingredients	*Directions*
1 tablespoon olive oil	*1* In a 4-quart saucepan, heat the olive oil over medium heat. Add the sliced onions to the pan and sauté for 3 minutes.
½ medium onion, thinly sliced	
¼ teaspoon cumin	
¼ teaspoon coriander	*2* Add the cumin, coriander, and curry powder to the saucepan with the onion and gently toast the spices for 1 minute. Stir in the chicken broth and chickpeas, and bring the soup to a boil. Reduce the heat and simmer for 10 minutes.
¼ teaspoon curry powder	
32 ounces chicken broth, low-sodium	
One 14.5 ounce can chickpeas, drained and rinsed	*3* Ladle the soup into 4 bowls. Serve with thin lemon slices and the chopped cilantro.
1 lemon, sliced thin	
¼ cup fresh cilantro, chopped	

Per serving: Calories 111 (From Fat 38); Fat 4g (Saturated 1g); Cholesterol 0mg; Sodium 160mg; Carbohydrate 13g (Dietary Fiber 3g); Protein 5g.

Vary It! For a heartier soup, add about ½ cup chopped carrots and celery.

Please pass the chickpeas

Popular for their nutty flavor and slight crunch, chickpeas are a food staple around the globe. When not eaten boiled, fried, or roasted, they're the main ingredient in many dishes you may have heard of, like hummus, falafel, Cuban bean soup, and *dhal* (a type of bean stew). Raw or roasted chickpeas can also be milled into gram flour, which is both gluten-free and protein-rich and used extensively in the cuisines of India, Pakistan, and Bangladesh.

One cup of cooked chickpeas has about 270 calories, 4 grams of fat, 12 grams of fiber, and 15 grams of protein, as well as a multitude of vitamins (thiamin, B6, folate, vitamins E, K, A, and C, riboflavin, and niacin) and minerals (calcium, magnesium, phosphorus, iron, zinc, and potassium).

For an extra nutritional punch, add chickpeas to salads, soups, stews, and stir fries. *Note:* If you're using canned chickpeas, be aware of the sodium content.

Prosciutto and Fresh Mozzarella Panini

Prep time: 10 min • **Cook time:** 8 min • **Yield:** 4 servings

Ingredients	Directions
Eight ½-inch thick slices of French or ciabatta bread **4 tablespoons olive oil**	**1** Heat a cast iron skillet over medium-high heat. While the skillet heats up, use a pastry brush to spread the olive oil evenly onto one side of each slice of French bread.
4 ounces fresh mozzarella, sliced into four 1-ounce slices **4 ounces prosciutto, thinly sliced**	**2** Assemble the sandwiches: On the unoiled side of four slices of bread, arrange the mozzarella, prosciutto, and basil leaves; place the remaining slices, oiled side up, on top.
8 fresh basil leaves	**3** Cook the sandwiches on one side until toasted, occasionally pressing down on the sandwich as it cooks to create a pressed-sandwich effect. Carefully turn the sandwiches over and toast the other side. Serve immediately.

Per serving: Calories 440 (From Fat 217); Fat 24g (Saturated 7g); Cholesterol 45mg; Sodium 1,185mg; Carbohydrate 36g (Dietary Fiber 2g); Protein 20g.

Tip: If you have a panini press, cook the sandwiches in that. Alternatively, simply cook the sandwiches as you would grilled cheese, foregoing the pressing altogether.

Making cheese add to your health, not to your hips

Cheese is a great source of healthy nutrients such as calcium, protein, phosphorus, zinc, vitamin A, riboflavin, and vitamin B-12. However, it also packs a lot of fat and calories. Going overboard with cheese can lead to weight gain and associated health problems such as heart disease or diabetes. The trick is to use the right types of cheese for a particular dish so that you can get a lot of flavor and avoid excessive calories and fat. Use these tips to enjoy cheese in a healthy way:

- When using a large amount of cheese in a recipe like lasagna, choose lower-fat cheeses like low-fat ricotta and part-skim mozzarella.

- Take advantage of part-skim mozzarella when eating cheese with crackers and bread.

- When cooking, use shredded cheese rather than chunks or slices. Most of the time, you end up using less cheese overall.

- With dishes like salads, eggs, or pastas, sprinkle a small amount of strong-flavored cheeses such as goat cheese, Parmesan, or feta. A little goes a long, long way with flavor.

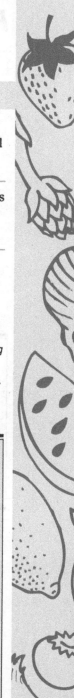

Fun Snacks

Who doesn't like snacks? Or perhaps a better question is "Who has the will-power to forego snacking?" The answer to both questions is "Practically no one." Fortunately, the keys to incorporating snacks into your diet are eating them in moderation and choosing healthy options.

If you follow these two guidelines, you can partake without guilt and even enjoy the good things that snacking can do for you. Healthy snacks keep your blood sugar levels from spiking and dropping (for more on the importance of blood sugar levels, refer to Chapter 5). They also help you avoid the cravings that lead to poor food choices.

When choosing your snacks, opt for things like seeds and nuts, low-fat dairy products, whole grains, and fruits and vegetables. To make the snack more satisfying (and maximize the nutritional punch), look to combine these things: a sliced apple with peanut butter, for example, or a whole grain pita with hummus. Consider the following recipes as your starter kit. Let them inspire your snack-time creations!

Making meals out of appetizers

Traditional Mediterranean cuisine is quite unique in that many people often don't have a main entrée, but instead they eat a series of small side dishes including a variety of different foods, such as meats, beans, vegetables, grains, and fruits. Lunch is the main meal, so dinner is often something light, such as a meze platter. Making dinner out of appetizers is easy because you have a good variety of foods to choose from. Nowadays, you can find many tapas restaurants sprouting up with this same idea of serving several small appetizers as a meal.

Fig Bundles

Prep time: 10 min • **Yield:** 32 servings

Ingredients	Directions
16 figs, sliced into halves 32 walnut halves	*1* Slice the figs in half (32 halves), and slice the prosciutto into 32 equal portions.
3 ounces prosciutto, thinly sliced 2 tablespoons honey	*2* Stuff 1 walnut half into each fig half and then wrap the fig half with prosciutto, securing it with a toothpick if desired. Repeat for the other fig halves.
	3 Place the fig bundles on a serving plate and drizzle with the honey before serving.

Per serving: Calories 43 (From Fat 14); Fat 2g (Saturated 0g); Cholesterol 2mg; Sodium 71mg; Carbohydrate 6g (Dietary Fiber 1g); Protein 3g.

Figs

Figs are a small fruit with a mild, sweet flavor. Most people think of figs as the sticky sweet spread in certain cookies or as dried figs, but if you've never eaten a fresh fig, you may be pleasantly surprised by its milder, less-sweet taste. Figs are ready to pick during the summer months in warm climates such as California. Fresh figs may not be easy to find in your local grocery store or farmers' market, but don't worry; you can order fresh figs and have them sent to your door from Passion Fruit Farms (http://www.figlady.com/).

Here's what you need to know about buying, storing, and eating fresh figs:

✔ Because they're so delicate, finding a perfectly ripe, unblemished fig is nearly impossible. But don't despair. Figs that have slightly wrinkled flesh are fine, as long as they're still plump. Similarly, ones whose skins have split are fine as well, as long as no juice is oozing from the split.

✔ To eat figs, simply remove the stem and pop them whole into your mouth. The flesh is sweet and chewy, and the edible seeds are crunchy.

✔ Figs spoil quickly, so plan on using them within a day or two of buying them. They store best at room temperature.

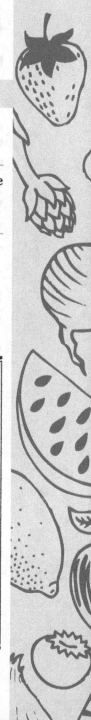

White Bean Dip

Prep time: 10 min • **Yield:** 6 servings

Ingredients	*Directions*
One 15-ounce can white beans, drained and rinsed	*1* Place the white beans, basil, artichoke hearts (if using), garlic, lemon juice, lemon zest, and olive oil into a food processor and pulse until the mixture is coarsely chopped.
½ cup fresh basil	
½ cup artichoke hearts packed in water, drained (optional)	
1 garlic clove	*2* Add salt and pepper to taste and serve the dip with pita chips, crackers, or fresh vegetables.
1 tablespoon lemon juice	
1 teaspoon lemon zest	
3 tablespoons extra virgin olive oil	
Salt and pepper to taste	

Per serving: Calories 102 (From Fat 60); Fat 7g (Saturated 1g); Cholesterol 0mg; Sodium 76mg; Carbohydrate 8g (Dietary Fiber 2g); Protein 3g.

Finding the perfect bean

The wide variety of available beans can be confusing and intimidating, so here's a breakdown of various kinds of beans with their distinct flavors and common uses:

- *Black beans* taste slightly sweet and are a great addition to salads, casseroles, soups, burritos, and dips.

- *Cannellini beans* offer a mild flavor and are common in Italian cooking. They work well in soups, stews, and casseroles.

- *Chickpeas,* with their nutty flavor and tougher texture, are great in casseroles and stews or with couscous or hummus.

- *Fava beans* have a nutty flavor and are often included in stews and side dishes.

- *Great Northern beans* are large, white beans with a mild flavor. You find them most often in soups, stews, and casseroles.

- *Lima beans* are green-colored beans that offer a mild, earthy flavor. They're great alone, warmed up as a side dish, or in soups and stews.

- *Pinto beans* are brown/orange beans with a rich, earthy flavor. You find pintos in foods like refried beans, burritos, or rice and beans.

- *Red kidney beans* are — you guessed it — red, kidney-shaped beans with a meaty flavor. They're perfect tossed on a salad or in soups or stews.

- *Soybeans* are full-flavored, and they're great as a warm side dish or used in soups.

Apricot Canapes

Prep time: 5 min • **Yield:** 1 serving

Ingredients	*Directions*
3 fresh apricot halves	***1*** Place the apricot halves on a serving plate. Spoon 1 teaspoon of goat cheese onto each half, followed by a basil leaf, and topped with ½ teaspoon of crushed almonds. Serve.
3 teaspoons crumbled goat cheese	
3 fresh basil leaves	
1½ teaspoon crushed almonds	

Per serving: Calories 67 (From Fat 34); Fat 4g (Saturated 1g); Cholesterol 9mg; Sodium 34mg; Carbohydrate 6g (Dietary Fiber 1g); Protein 2g.

Tip: These canapes make an easy snack or appetizer for your next party!

Nutty for nuts

A bowl of nuts with a nutcracker is a common appearance on countertops across the Mediterranean region, especially during the holidays. The early Romans considered the walnut food for the gods and also commonly used its oil. Italians mastered the art of roasting chestnuts at Christmastime, bringing a tradition that's told in songs and stories around the world.

Having a bowl of walnuts or roasted chestnuts on your counter is a wonderful snack any time of year for visitors and family coming and going. Nuts provide healthy fats to your diet, helping you reduce your risk of heart disease. But remember: Everything in moderation; nuts also have a lot of calories, which can add up quickly. Enjoy an ounce or two of nuts each day to help keep your heart healthy. Here are a few ways to enjoy nuts:

✔ Sprinkle some walnuts, almonds, or pistachios on your salads.

✔ Have an ounce of your favorite nuts as a snack with a piece of fruit.

✔ Set out some nuts with a nutcracker for family and friends at parties, celebrations, or holidays.

✔ Add toasted almonds to green beans and toasted walnuts to asparagus.

✔ Add any kind of toasted nut (almonds, walnuts, pecans, hazelnuts, and so on) to your oatmeal.

✔ Make your own salad dressings, using peanut or walnut oil as the base.

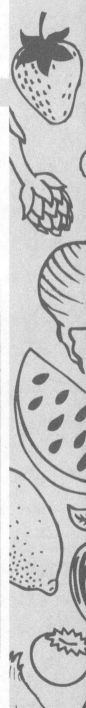

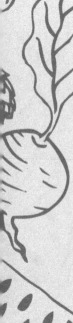
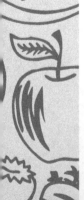

Minty Yogurt Dip with Fresh Berries

Prep time: 8 min • **Yield:** 2 servings

Ingredients	Directions
1 cup low-fat vanilla Greek yogurt	**1** Place the yogurt and mint leaves in a food processor or blender and blend until smooth.
2 to 3 fresh mint leaves	
1 cup fresh berries (any you like)	**2** Divide the berries into two bowls and add ½ cup of the dip on top. Serve.

Per serving: Calories 139 (From Fat 15); Fat 2g (Saturated 1g); Cholesterol 6mg; Sodium 45mg; Carbohydrate 23g (Dietary Fiber 1g); Protein 10g.

Berry delicious and healthy

Berries, such as strawberries, blueberries, and blackberries, are sweet, make the perfect quick dessert, and provide powerful health benefits. They're loaded with different nutrients, including antioxidants, vitamins, minerals, and phytochemicals, which all help lower your risk of diseases such as heart disease and certain cancers.

The only downside to berries is that they can spoil quickly. The best way to get berries is to pick them or to buy them at a local farmers' market. When buying berries at your grocery store, make sure the berries have no soft spots or mold for best quality.

Try some of these ideas for ways to include berries through out your day:

✔ Add berries to salads or to cereals.

✔ Infuse teas, water, and other drinks with fresh berries.

✔ Dip fresh strawberries in chocolate sauce.

✔ Combine dried berries, nuts, and sunflower or pumpkin seeds for a quick trail mix.

✔ Add a dollop of whipped cream to a bowl of your favorite berries. Top with some pistachios, slivered almonds, or shaved dark chocolate.

✔ Add fresh berries to vanilla or chocolate frozen yogurt.

✔ Mix your favorite berries with chocolate pudding.

✔ Blend berries, banana, and yogurt to make a fruit smoothie. Freeze your fruit smoothie with popsicle sticks to make a delicious frozen treat!

Enjoying More-Substantial Fare: Dinners

Lunch is the big meal in Mediterranean countries. Dinner is a relatively small affair. Not so in the typical American diet. When families are busy and workdays are long, a relaxing meal at the end of the day is a well-deserved — and needed — break. Make sure it's a healthy one, too.

Making animal protein a costar rather than the main attraction

Chances are you're accustomed to the meat being the star of your plate. The recipes in this section challenge you to think about animal-based protein sources a bit differently: as an accompanying star rather than the headliner. In the Mediterranean, meat, poultry, and even seafood portions are typically small, supporting parts of the meal rather than the main dish. This smaller serving means individuals in the Mediterranean consume less animal fat. They fill that extra plate space with plant-based proteins such as beans and lentils. This way of eating may seem a bit odd, but give it a try. You'll notice the health benefits after a short while. For more advice on how to change up the components on your plate, refer to Chapter 1.

As you prepare the chicken and seafood recipes in this chapter, remember the following:

- ✔ Chicken can carry *salmonella,* a type of bacteria that can cause foodborne illness. Always cook your chicken through — to 165 degrees — so that no pink is left in the center. Verify the temperature by placing a kitchen thermometer into the thickest part of the meat and make sure that it isn't touching any bones.

- ✔ When you cook with any animal protein, be it fish, shellfish, chicken, beef, pork, or any other, be certain to wash your hands and work surfaces thoroughly with antibacterial soap. Don't forget to always discard marinades after using.

Staying apprised of safety info related to fish and shellfish

Eating fish is an important part of a healthy diet; fish provides a lean source of protein and is rich in omega-3 fatty acids, which are important for heart health and mental health. Consuming fish several times a week is one of the

Mediterranean population's healthy habits. Nevertheless, you need to follow certain guidelines to ensure that you avoid any health issues potentially related to seafood.

First, make sure that you cook shellfish thoroughly. Shellfish, especially oysters, clams, mussels, and scallops, can carry bacteria called *Vibrio Vulnificus*. This nasty microbe can multiply even when refrigerated. The bacteria are usually destroyed by the immune systems of healthy people, but that is not always the case, and the result can be diarrhea, vomiting, blistering skin, and even, occasionally, death. Fortunately, you can easily avoid putting yourself at risk by making sure you cook your shellfish thoroughly to destroy the bacteria. Cook scallops until they're white and firm and mollusks until the shells open. Throw away any that don't open.

Second, remember that all seafood contains traces of *mercury*, a neurotoxin that accumulates in streams and oceans from industrial pollution. Babies and small children are at the highest risk because mercury levels may exceed the safety limits for their small weight. For the average healthy adult, limiting your intake of the high-mercury fish listed here can keep you pretty safe:

- Avoid shark, swordfish, king mackerel (kingfish), and tilefish because they contain high levels of mercury.
- Choose light canned tuna as opposed to albacore canned tuna because the former has less mercury.
- Consume up to 12 ounces per week of lower-mercury seafood, including shrimp, salmon, pollock, and catfish.
- Check your local advisories on any local fish caught in lakes and streams. If no advisories are available, eat up to 6 ounces per week of such local fish with no additional fish (of any kind) that week.

These guidelines are especially important for pregnant women, nursing moms, women who may become pregnant, and small children. Refer to Chapter 12 for more information related to safe consumption of fish and seafood.

Eating pasta responsibly

Pasta is one of those foods that can be part of a healthy diet or can become a not-so-healthy problem. People in the United States and Canada typically eat pasta in large portion sizes and with high-calorie sauces, which can contribute to weight gain. Keeping pasta healthy is a fine line, but if you stick to the following tips, you can enjoy your pasta, keep your figure, and stay in good health:

✔ **Watch your portion sizes closely.** Pasta is most commonly a side dish in the Mediterranean. Keep your portion sizes at between a half cup and a full cup to avoid eating too many calories and to keep your blood sugar stable. This strategy helps you stay trim and keeps your heart healthy.

✔ **Avoid eating heavy entrees with heavy side dishes.** If you're eating pasta with a heavier, higher-fat and higher-calorie sauce (such as a béchamel sauce), make sure the rest of your meal is on the light side, like a simple salad.

✔ **Add a little protein.** If you're eating an entree that includes pasta, make sure you have some protein as well. This addition may mean including seafood or meat in your pasta or having nuts and beans in a side salad. Adding protein provides a more balanced meal and helps maintain stable blood sugar.

✔ **Don't fill up on just pasta.** You don't want to eat a large amount of pasta at once. Instead, load up your small portion of pasta with proteins and lots of fresh vegetables so that you still feel like you have a hearty entree. Imagine a half cup of pasta with tomato sauce on a plate compared to a half cup of pasta mixed with broccoli, carrots, and chicken. The latter makes a larger volume of food without filling up an entire dish with pasta.

✔ **Don't overcook your pasta.** In Italy, pasta is always cooked *al dente*, firm to the teeth but tender for chewing. Cooking your pasta al dente is actually a healthier way to eat because doing so gives the pasta a lower glycemic index (the pasta doesn't spike your blood sugar as quickly).

Grilled Tuna with Avocado and Citrus Salsa

Prep time: 20 min • **Cook time:** 12 min • **Yield:** 4 servings

Ingredients	Directions
¼ cup olive oil	**1** In a shallow baking pan, combine the olive oil, lemon zest, garlic, and parsley. Mix the marinade well and season with salt and pepper to taste. Add the tuna steaks and marinate for 15 minutes.
1 lemon, zested and cut into wedges	
2 cloves garlic, minced	
¼ cup curly or Italian parsley, finely chopped	**2** While the tuna marinates, heat the grill over medium-high heat. In a small bowl, mix together the avocado, orange and grapefruit segments, jalapeno, red onion, and parsley. Season the salsa with salt and pepper to taste.
Salt and pepper to taste	
Four 4-ounce tuna steaks	
1 avocado, diced	**3** Grill the tuna steaks for 4 to 6 minutes on each side, or until slightly pink on the inside. Serve the grilled tuna with the salsa immediately.
1 orange, segmented and chopped	
1 grapefruit, segmented and chopped	
1 jalapeno, minced	
¼ red onion, minced	

Per serving: Calories 316 (From Fat 136); Fat 15g (Saturated 3g); Cholesterol 42mg; Sodium 194mg; Carbohydrate 19g (Dietary Fiber 6g); Protein 28g.

Getting schooled on fish

When you can't find the kind of fish your recipes ask for, consider these substitutes:

Calls for	*Substitute with*
Cod	Snapper, mahi-mahi, walleye, or perch
Halibut	Grouper, cod, salmon, tilapia, or snapper
Tuna	Wahoo, halibut, salmon, or trout
Salmon	Trout, whitefish, or striped bass
Sea bass	Tuna, halibut, or trout

Swiss Chard and Chicken Gratin

Prep time: 25 min • **Cook time:** 35 min • **Yield:** 6 servings

Ingredients	*Directions*
1 tablespoon olive oil	*1* Preheat the oven to 400 degrees.
½ medium onion, thinly sliced	
4 slices bacon, chopped	*2* In a heavy skillet, heat the olive oil over medium-high heat. Add the onions and chopped bacon, and sauté for 4 minutes, or until the bacon crisps up. Lower the heat to medium, add the garlic and sauté for 1 minute. Add the stems from the chard and sauté for 2 minutes. Add the greens and sauté until slightly wilted. Remove the skillet from the heat, stir in the cooked chicken, and then place the mixture into an 8-x-8-inch baking pan.
4 cloves garlic, chopped	
8 cups Swiss chard, stems separated from leaves	
2 cups cooked, chopped chicken breast	
8 ounces goat cheese	*3* Place the goat cheese in the skillet, heat over medium heat, stirring constantly until the cheese is melted. Stir in the half-and-half; continue to stir until the mixture becomes saucy and then add the Parmesan cheese. Stir until the Parmesan melts.
1 cup half-and-half or milk	
¾ cup Parmesan cheese, grated	
1 cup bread crumbs	*4* Pour the cheese sauce over the greens, top evenly with the bread crumbs, and bake for 30 minutes. When done, allow the dish to sit for a few minutes before serving.

Per serving: *Calories 412 (From Fat 213); Fat 24g (Saturated 12g); Cholesterol 115mg; Sodium 708mg; Carbohydrate 20g (Dietary Fiber 2g); Protein 32g.*

Chicken facts

To get the most flavor from your chicken and make the best choices, keep in mind that each part of the chicken contains varying degrees of fat. The white meat from the breast is the leanest cut, followed by the thigh (as long as the skin is removed). The wings and legs are higher in fat (they have about as much fat as some cuts of beef).

Also, although removing the skin can lower the fat content, you can do so after cooking to create a juicier and tastier poultry dish that is still considered low fat. In addition, chicken fat consists of mostly good-for-you monounsaturated and polyunsaturated fats, so eating some dark chicken meat once in a while isn't as harmful to your health as you may have thought. Just watch your portion size (2 to 3 ounces) and don't deep fry it.

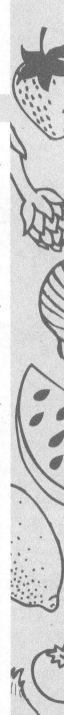

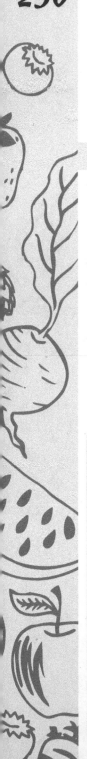

Chickpea and Lemon Parsley Salad with Grilled Pita

Prep time: 10 min • **Cook time:** 3 min • **Yield:** 4 servings

Ingredients	Directions
Two 14.5-ounce cans chickpeas, drained and rinsed	**1** In a serving bowl, mix together the chickpeas, lemon zest, lemon juice, parsley, cucumber, and olive oil. Stir the chickpea salad together and season with salt and pepper to taste.
1 lemon, zested and juiced	
1 cup curly or Italian parsley, finely chopped	**2** Heat a cast iron skillet or griddle over medium-high heat. Toast the pita bread on each side until slightly browned, about 2 to 3 minutes. Divide the salad onto 4 plates and serve each with a toasted pita.
1 medium cucumber, diced	
¼ cup olive oil	
Salt and pepper to taste	
4 pita breads	

Per serving: Calories 412 (From Fat 143); Fat 16g (Saturated 2g); Cholesterol 0mg; Sodium 522mg; Carbohydrate 56g (Dietary Fiber 7g); Protein 12g.

Keeping your recipes fresh: Cooking with lemons

Lemon juice provides a nice, light citrus flavor and can also enhance the overall flavor of a meal. By using lemons, you can use much less salt and fewer added fats without sacrificing flavor. And that's not to mention the health benefits: Lemons are high in vitamin C and other phytonutrients, which act as antioxidants to help prevent damage to your cells. Here are a few tips for using lemons in your cooking:

✔ To get the most juice, juice lemons at room temperature instead of cold and roll them firmly on the counter before juicing to break up the pulp.

✔ When making a recipe that calls for lemon juice, go the extra mile and fill an ice cube tray with lemon juice so that you can freeze portions for easy use in later recipes.

✔ Use a few squeezes of lemon juice on your salad and use a third to half less salad dressing to save some fat and calories. (**Note:** This tip only works with vinaigrettes that aren't lemon-based.)

✔ Add lemon juice to sliced apples and pears to keep them from browning.

✔ Use lemon juice to tenderize meats.

✔ Add lemon juice to cooked rice to make it fluffier and enhance the flavor.

Tortellini with Tomatoes and Spinach

Prep time: 10 min • **Cook time:** 15 min • **Yield:** 4 servings

Ingredients	Directions
One 7-ounce package of dry or fresh cheese tortellini	**1** Cook the tortellini according to the package directions.
¼ cup extra virgin olive oil	
Juice of one lemon	**2** While the tortellini cooks, whisk together in a small bowl the olive oil, lemon juice, vinegar, zest, and salt. Set the dressing aside.
1 tablespoon white wine vinegar	
1 tablespoon finely grated lemon zest	**3** Drain the cooked tortellini and pour it into a medium-sized bowl. Add the tomatoes, spinach, and basil, and toss the pasta with the lemon dressing.
½ teaspoon salt	
1 Roma tomato, chopped	**4** Add the cheese (if using) to the pasta mixture and toss gently. Divide the tortellini among the bowls, add salt and pepper to taste, and serve.
4 cups fresh baby spinach	
½ cup fresh basil, cut into strips	
¼ cup grated Parmesan cheese (optional)	
Salt and pepper to taste	

Per serving: Calories 289 (From Fat 153); Fat 17g (Saturated 4g); Cholesterol 21mg; Sodium 524mg; Carbohydrate 27g (Dietary Fiber 2g); Protein 8g.

Tip: Add more or less of the lemon juice and zest, depending on how much lemon flavor you enjoy.

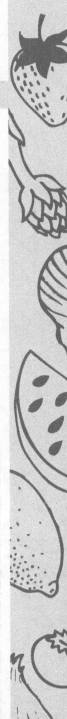

Shrimp, Tomato, and Basil Pasta

Prep time: 12 min • **Cook time:** 22 min • **Yield:** 4 servings

Ingredients	Directions
1 tablespoon olive oil 2 garlic cloves, peeled and minced 1 pound Roma tomatoes, coarsely chopped, or one 16-ounce can diced plum tomatoes ½ cup fresh basil leaves, coarsely chopped ¼ teaspoon crushed red pepper flakes 1½ pounds medium shrimp, peeled and deveined with tails removed ½ pound linguine pasta Salt and pepper to taste	**1** In a large skillet, heat the olive oil over medium heat. Add the garlic and sauté for about 1 minute, allowing the garlic to lightly brown. Add the tomatoes, basil, and crushed red pepper, and simmer for 12 minutes. **2** Add the shrimp and cook an additional 3 to 4 minutes, until the shrimp is opaque and cooked through. Remove the shrimp from the skillet and set aside. **3** Meanwhile, cook the pasta in a large sauce pan, according to the package directions. When done, drain the pasta and return it to the pan. Add the cooked shrimp and tomato sauce, season with salt and pepper to taste, and toss. Serve immediately.

Per serving: Calories 348 (From Fat 56); Fat 6g (Saturated 1g); Cholesterol 161mg; Sodium 877mg; Carbohydrate 48g (Dietary Fiber 4g); Protein 26g.

Cooking pasta to perfection

The key to cooking pasta is to make sure it's cooked al dente and not overly soft. Here are some tips for cooking great, healthy pasta:

✔ Be sure to use a large pot with a good amount of water (usually at least 3 quarts) so that the pasta cooks evenly and doesn't stick together.

✔ Don't add oil, which actually makes your pasta too slippery for the sauce to adhere well.

✔ Stir the cooking pasta occasionally to make sure it doesn't stick to the bottom.

✔ For more flavor, add salt to your pasta water while it's boiling.

✔ For most pastas, don't rinse after draining. Just toss it directly with the sauce. Rinsing decreases the flavor and makes the pasta less sticky.

✔ Rinse noodles (such as manicotti or lasagna) that you're going to stuff or layer. Doing so makes the pasta easier to handle and halts any further cooking.

Diving into Desserts

Serving up a variety of great desserts is common practice on the Mediterranean coast. So how do the people who live there stay heart healthy and manage their weight? Moderation is the secret.

For weekly dessert treats, Mediterranean residents often eat just plain fruit or a small cookie such as biscotti. You also see fruit desserts lightly sweetened with a little sugar or honey. The more-robust desserts the region is famous for, such as baklava, are reserved for special occasions like holidays and festivals. Some desserts are served for a specific symbolic meaning, such as desserts made with eggs at Easter.

As with all Mediterranean-style cooking, the dessert menu often includes an abundance of the region's commonly grown foods, such as nuts, apricots, dates, lemons, and oranges.

In this section, you can find a variety of desserts. Many of these recipes certainly make the cut for a weekly treat because they're lower in fat, calories, and sugar than many store-bought desserts.

How many nuts are enough?

Nuts are widely used in Mediterranean cuisine, making a healthy, satisfying snack and adding wonderful flavor to many recipes. You want to be careful though with how much you eat. Although they contain healthy fats, they still can add up in calories, which means potential for weight gain. A serving size of nuts is typically about 1 ounce, which breaks down to the following for the specific type of nut:

- Almonds: 20 to 24
- Brazil nuts: 6 to 8
- Cashews: 16 to 18
- Hazelnuts: 18 to 20
- Macadamias: 10 to 12
- Peanuts: 28
- Pecans: 15 halves
- Pine nuts: 150 to 157
- Pistachios: 45 to 47
- Walnuts: 14 halves

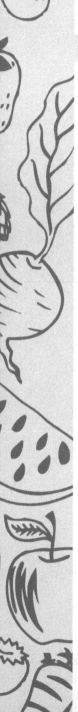

Chocolate Avocado Cake

Prep time: 15 min • **Cook time:** 40 min • **Yield:** 12 servings

Ingredients	Directions
3 cups all-purpose flour, plus enough to dust pan	**1** Preheat the oven to 350 degrees. Spray a 9-x-9-inch baking pan with cooking spray and lightly coat it with all-purpose flour.
⅓ cup unsweetened cocoa powder	
½ teaspoon salt	**2** In a large mixing bowl, whisk together the flour, cocoa powder, salt, and baking soda. Set aside.
2 teaspoons baking soda	
½ cup soft avocado, mashed	**3** In another large mixing bowl, mix the avocado, water, and vanilla. Add the sugar and oil to the wet ingredients and mix well.
2 cups water	
2 teaspoon vanilla extract	
2 cups granulated sugar	**4** Add the wet ingredients to dry ingredients and blend until the batter is smooth. Pour the batter into the prepared baking pan.
¼ cup vegetable oil	
½ cup powdered sugar	**5** Bake the cake for 30 to 40 minutes. Then remove from the oven and allow the cake to cool completely. To serve, dust the cake lightly with powdered sugar.

Per serving: Calories 327 (From Fat 60); Fat 7g (Saturated 1g); Cholesterol 0mg; Sodium 309mg; Carbohydrate 65g (Dietary Fiber 2g); Protein 4g.

Vary It! You can replace the powdered sugar with cream cheese frosting.

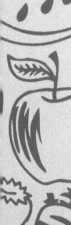

Semolina and Coconut Cake with Almonds

Prep time: 20 min, plus sitting time • **Cook time:** 30 min • **Yield:** 9 servings

Ingredients	Directions
2 cups semolina flour	*1* Preheat the oven to 350 degrees. Lightly coat a 9-inch pie pan with cooking spray.
1 cup shredded coconut, unsweetened	
1½ teaspoons baking powder	*2* In a large mixing bowl, whisk together the semolina flour, coconut, baking powder, and sugar. Drizzle the water into the flour and mix, using your fingers, until the mixture resembles crumbs. Add the milk and stir together until mixed completely.
½ cup sugar	
¼ cup warm water	
1½ cups low-fat milk	
Sugar Syrup (see the following recipe)	*3* Spread the dough into the pie pan and bake for 20 minutes. While the cake cooks, prepare the Sugar Syrup (see the following recipe) and set aside until ready to use.
9 almonds, blanched	
	4 Remove the pie from the oven and score 9 pie slices on the surface while the cake is hot and slightly under-cooked. Top each piece with a blanched almond. Return the cake to the oven and bake for an additional 10 minutes, or until golden brown. Pour the Sugar Syrup over the cake, allowing the syrup to soak in for few hours before serving.

Sugar Syrup

1 cup sugar	*1* Mix the sugar and water in a 2-quart saucepan and heat over medium-high heat until the sugar is dissolved and the mixture is slightly thickened.
1 cup water	
½ lemon, juiced	
1 teaspoon orange blossom water or rose water	*2* Remove the sugar water from the heat and add a squeeze of lemon and the orange blossom or rose water. Allow the syrup to cool until ready to use.

Per serving: Calories 505 (From Fat 211); Fat 24g (Saturated 5g); Cholesterol 2mg; Sodium 112mg; Carbohydrate 68g (Dietary Fiber 2g); Protein 7g.

Dark Chocolate Almond Bites

Prep time: 30 min • **Yield:** 32 servings

Ingredients	*Directions*
4 ounces dark chocolate	*1* Line two baking sheets with parchment paper and set aside.
¼ cup heavy whipping cream	
¼ teaspoon instant espresso granules	*2* In a double boiler, melt the dark chocolate. Whisk in the heavy whipping cream and expresso powder and remove the pan from the heat.
2 cups shaved almonds	
1 orange, zested	*3* Gently stir the almonds and orange zest into the melted chocolate. With a kitchen spoon, measure out 1 tablespoon of dark chocolate–covered almonds onto the parchment paper. Repeat until the almond mixture is gone. You'll have about 32 stacks.
	4 Chill the bites in the refrigerator for at least 1 hour before serving. Store the chocolate bites in the refrigerator in an airtight container.

Tip: Place additional layers of parchment between the layers of chocolate to prevent the bites from sticking to one another during storage.

Per serving: Calories 59 (From Fat 42); Fat 5g (Saturated 1g); Cholesterol 3mg; Sodium 2mg; Carbohydrate 4g (Dietary Fiber 1g); Protein 1g.

Making room for almonds

Almonds have a lot of good things to recommend them as part of your healthy diet. First (and most important), they taste great. Enjoy them alone, add slivers to rice or vegetable dishes, toss them in salads, use almond flour in pancakes, and make shakes with almond milk. Second, they offer all sorts of health benefits:

✔ The fat in almonds is the monounsaturated kind (refer to Chapter 2 for more on healthy fats).

✔ They're packed with vitamin E and contain large amounts of phytonutrients, which are heart healthy.

✔ Studies indicate that they may play a role in weight loss, lowering cholesterol, and reducing the risk of heart disease.

For all the good things almonds include, one thing they aren't a good source for is omega-3 fatty acids. Look to other nuts, like walnuts, for those.

Grapes and Pistachios over Greek Yogurt

Prep time: 5 min • **Yield:** 4 servings

Ingredients	Directions
2 cups whole fat or 2% Greek yogurt	*1* Place ½ cup of the Greek yogurt into each of four bowls.
2 cups purple grapes, sliced in half	
¼ cup pistachios, chopped	*2* In a mixing bowl, combine the grapes, pistachios, honey, and lemon juice. Stir until combined.
4 tablespoons honey	
½ lemon, juiced	*3* Evenly top the Greek yogurt with the grape salad and garnish with mint prior to serving.
¼ cup fresh mint, chopped	

Per serving: Calories 238 (From Fat 53); Fat 6g (Saturated 2g); Cholesterol 8mg; Sodium 75mg; Carbohydrate 39g (Dietary Fiber 2g); Protein 12g.

Adding a touch of fruit to sweeten your meal

Using fruit in desserts (from cakes to cookies) is common practice in the Mediterranean. Actually, fruit itself is often a simple dessert, which is another key to the health benefits found in the Mediterranean lifestyle.

Getting in the habit of eating a little fruit when you have a sweet tooth is a great wellness strategy. Eating abundant amounts of fruit means consuming more healthy nutrients such as vitamins, antioxidants, and fiber, which help you lower your risk of certain diseases.

Fruit-filled desserts are more satisfying; lower in calories, fat, and sugar; and richer in healthy nutrients than the processed sweets you can pick up at the store.

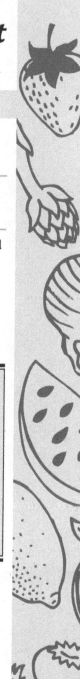

Part V
The Part of Tens

For a bonus Mediterranean diet part of tens chapter, head online to www.dummies.com/extras/mediterraneandiet.

In this part . . .

✔ Incorporate a variety of spices to not only enhance the flavor of anything you prepare but also maximize the health benefits associated with the Mediterranean diet.

✔ Read about the groundbreaking studies that show the link between diet and health in general and that demonstrate a direction connection between the Mediterranean diet and heart health.

✔ Discover easy ways to incorporate the key principles of the Mediterranean diet into your current diet and lifestyle, even if you're not quite ready to fully embrace the diet itself.

Chapter 17

A Taste of the Mediterranean: Top Ten Herbs and Spices

In This Chapter

▶ Highlighting the herbs and spices popular to the Mediterranean cuisine

▶ Adding a dash of Mediterranean flavor to any meal

*H*erbs, spices, and lots of flavor — those are the things you'll discover when you partake of Mediterranean cuisine. For thousands of years, herbs and spices have been incorporated into Mediterranean dishes to add flavor. What we know now is that these additions boost flavor without adding a significant amount of calories, sodium, or fat. In fact, herbs and spices are so essential to the cuisine, that they've earned a place in the Mediterranean food guide pyramid alongside fruits, vegetables, olive oil, grains, seeds, nuts, and legumes (refer to Chapter 1).

Herbs and spices not only spice up your dish for the benefit of your taste buds, but they also pack a nutritional punch! They contain a range of phytonutrients and antioxidants and, by type, offer up various health benefits. So go ahead, take a simple cue from the Mediterranean cuisine and experiment with a variety of herbs and spices to reap the benefits.

Basil

Basil, or sweet basil as used in Italian or Greek cuisine, comes from the Greek word for *king*, and many culinary experts consider it the "king of herbs" because of the wide variety of uses.

Basil is best (and most commonly) used fresh for the fullest flavor and clove scent. Also, cooking and drying destroy basil's flavor.

Herbs versus spices

You may be wondering what, exactly, is the difference between an herb and a spice. Well, both come from plants. The differences relate to where on the plant they come from: the leaf or the other parts. These quick explanations should clear things up:

✔ **Herbs** are the leaves from non-woody plants. Whether fresh or dried, common herbs are basil, chives, mint, oregano, parsley, rosemary, sage, and thyme. So the thyme you grow is an herb. So is the dried thyme you have in your spice cupboard. You can buy herbs fresh or dried (which saves you money!). Use 1 teaspoon of the dried version for about 1 tablespoon of the fresh variety.

✔ **Spices** are produced from any part of the plant except the leaves (root, bark, flowers, and fruits), and are typically bought dried or in clove version (such as garlic). Common spices include cinnamon (bark), cloves (flower bud), ginger (root), nutmeg (seed), and pepper (fruit).

All of which begs the question: What is salt? (A mineral, in case you're curious.)

Here are some of the many ways you'll see fresh basil leaves used:

✔ Atop a slice of pizza or pasta dishes

✔ Minced into raw salads (basil can be used interchangeably with mint)

✔ Added to soups and hot dishes after they're removed from the heat

✔ Blended into uncooked condiments like vinaigrettes, mayonnaise, infused oils, and hummus.

✔ As the prominently featured herb in pesto sauces (made with crushed garlic, pine nuts, olive oil, and Parmesan cheese).

 Basil may be your best friend as you age and your joints succumb to arthritis and inflammation. It contains an essential oil, *eugenol,* that blocks the enzymes that cause swelling. Basil also contains powerful flavonoids such as zeaxanthin, which protects your eyes from UV rays and can help slow age-related macular disease.

Cilantro

The Spanish word for *coriander,* cilantro specifically refers to the leaves on the coriander plant. People either love or hate cilantro in dishes. But the Mediterranean diet loves this herb, which is rich in phytonutrients. Use it to add a punch of flavor and crisp texture to salads, bean dishes, soups, and salsas. In Spain, cilantro is often blended into sauces made to accompany meat and fish dishes. In America, too, sales of cilantro rise over Super Bowl weekend and Cinco de Mayo, times when guacamole and salsas are popular.

Whether you love or hate cilantro may actually be determined by your genes. According to studies, your DNA may determine whether cilantro smells good or bad (or, as Julia Child, a cilantro hater, has proclaimed, has a soapy or "dead" taste).

If you've never been a fan, try crushing cilantro, which removes the aroma, before you use it in cooking.

Cinnamon

You may automatically associate cinnamon as the go-to spice when you're making sweet baked goods like coffee cake, cinnamon rolls, puddings, or baked apples. Maybe you sprinkle it atop fruit or add it to your oatmeal. The same is true in Mediterranean cuisine: Consider the traditional dessert baklava a case in point. But in the Mediterranean, cinnamon is used in more savory dishes, as well, such as a Moroccan rub for a meat dish.

Cinnamon — available in stick or powdered form — has been found in research to help people with diabetes control their blood glucose levels. It also has anti-clotting and anti-inflammatory properties due to its compound coumarin.

That being said, cinnamon should not be considered a replacement for any medical treatment in these areas. If you have diabetes or are taking prescription anti-clotting medications, check with your doctor before using cinnamon in large quantities (basically more than a sprinkling a few times per day) in your diet.

Dill

Commonly found in traditional Greek *tzatziki,* or yogurt sauce, dill is a great source of antioxidants and calcium (about 60 mg per ounce), helping reduce your risk for bone-related disease. Often, you'll find that you toast dill seeds before using them in recipes (the heat brings out their aroma and flavor). They taste similar to caraway seeds or fennel.

If you're worried about how and when to use dill, just relax! An agent in dill weed called *carvone* has a calming effect and may help reduce intestinal distress, too. If that's not calming enough, here are some ideas to ease your mind:

✔ Chop dill into a cucumber yogurt dip or mustard sauce

✔ Sprinkle chopped dill into salads or over rice or egg dishes

✔ Add dill seeds when pickling cucumbers

✔ Use dill as a garnish on soups

✔ Pair dill with garlic or rosemary to season potatoes

Garlic

Garlic comes in many forms — fresh as a clove, dried, minced, and in powder — and has been found to have a multitude of health benefits, too! Worried about bad breath? Maybe this info will help you change your tune. Research out of UCLA found that taking 1,200 mg of aged garlic extract per day can be a powerful barrier to plaque build-up, can help reduce cholesterol and blood pressure, and can lower the risk for cardiac events and heart disease. Also, the phytonutrients responsible for garlic's odor, *allicin* and *dialyll disulphide*, have antibacterial and antiviral properties that can help protect against infections, ranging from the common cold to cancer.

Keeping herbs and spices fresh

Herbs and spices can be pretty pricey, so you want to make sure that what you have doesn't go to waste. Even dried herbs and spices can go bad (within six months to a year). Follow these suggestions to maximize both the nutrient and taste benefits:

✔ **If possible, buy herbs and spices in small amounts, especially for those you don't use frequently.** Specialized spice shops, ethnic markets, and some larger grocery stores enable you to buy small amounts of spices.

✔ **Clean out your spice rack regularly.** If you're not sure whether a spice is near the end of its life, take a sniff. Spices should be aromatic. If you have to sniff hard to get a whiff or smell something in addition to the spice itself, toss it. Ground cloves, for example, should smell only like ground cloves.

✔ **If you can't use fresh herbs right away, freeze them to minimize waste and extend their shelf life.** Just wash, pat dry, place in a resealable freezer bag, press out the air, and toss in the freezer. You don't need to thaw them before using. For thin herbs (like chives), chop them before freezing.

Note: Pre-bought seasonings contain both herbs and spices, but they may also contain some undesirable ingredients like sodium. Always be sure to check the label to see what you're getting.

Garlic is oh so versatile. Here are some of my favorite ways to eat it:

- ✔ Mixed with hummus to use as a dip or sandwich spread
- ✔ Sautéed with olive oil and mixed into a side dish like spinach
- ✔ Added to a sauce or marinade to be used with chicken and fish
- ✔ Baked into whole wheat garlic bread
- ✔ Roasted whole to eat the cloves on their own, to whip into mashed potatoes, or to spread on whole wheat bread

Lemon

Okay, you're right, this isn't an herb or spice, but I'd be remiss not to mention lemon when discussing the flavors of the Mediterranean. It's true that lemon falls into the fruit category but not one that you eat whole. Instead, the lemon's juice, rind, and zest are added to dishes to impart a sour and tart flavor. Nutritionally speaking, lemon is a great source of the powerful antioxidant vitamin C.

The countries of the Mediterranean make up lemon's major producers, and, boy, do the people in these regions like to use them: in pasta, in rice, and in fish dishes; as a main flavor in soups like *avgolemono* (a mixture of lemon juice, egg, and broth); squeezed over salads; paired with roasted veggies; added to baked goods; and as a cool summer treat (in lemon ices, for example).

Freeze freshly squeezed lemon juice in ice cube trays and store it in the freezer for later use. You can also keep lemon zest in an airtight container stored in a cool, dry place.

Mint

Think outside of the tea bag. Mint originated in the Mediterranean. Fresh mint is often used in dishes like *tabbouleh* (a salad made with cracked wheat and other ingredients), soups, rice, and bean dishes. It's chopped into sauces for lamb dishes and curries, is used in a yogurt sauce, and is added to punch up the flavor of just about anything: gelato, jellies, and gum to name just a few items. It also serves as a garnish to the plate.

The sweetly-flavored mint leaves like peppermint and spearmint have been used for medicinal purposes: as a decongestant and to a relieve digestive disorders and stomach cramps. Rich in vitamins A and C, mint also promotes eye health and gives your immune system a boost.

Fun Mediterranean fact! Mint is a symbol of hospitality in many cultures. In ancient Greece, it was rubbed onto dining room tables to welcome guests. Why not welcome mint into your diet, too?

Red Pepper Flakes

To really dial up the spice in your meal, add red pepper flakes. If you like spicy heat (as do many people of the Mediterranean), you'll have no problem applying these generously to any type of dish. Made from hot dried and crushed cayenne, bell, and ancho peppers, red pepper flakes are a good source of *capsaicin,* a component that fights inflammation and heart disease, and, studies suggest, can boost your metabolism.

If you aren't used to spicy food, go slowly with adding red pepper flakes to your diet. The more and more you use it, the more heat you'll be able to handle. Here are some suggestions:

- ✔ Grind flakes into powder for a dry rub on meat, fish, and vegetables
- ✔ Add the flakes to eggs or omelets to give breakfast a kick
- ✔ Sprinkle red pepper flakes over pasta, rice, or bean dishes, or on pizza
- ✔ Mix the flakes into dips, spreads, and salsas
- ✔ Use red pepper flakes to flavor stews, salads, and even desserts, especially rich, chocolate desserts!

Saffron

Most of the world's supply of saffron originates in the Mediterranean, Translated as "yellow" in Arabic, saffron lends a yellow-orange hue to dishes because of its natural carotenoid, *crocin.* Carotenoids, a precursor for vitamin A, are antioxidants that promote eye health, boost your immune system, and offer protection against cancer. Saffron adds a strong bitter, honey-like taste to rice and seafood dishes such as pilaf, paella, and bouillabaisse.

Although saffron is one of the most expensive spices, a little bit goes a long way. Just a pinch of threads provides enough for a recipe that serves four to six people. Before you can use it in cooking, you need to prepare the saffron from the threads. After taking a pinch, follow these steps:

1. **Crush the saffron threads with a mortar and pestle.**

2. **Soak the crushed saffron in a few tablespoons of hot water for at least 10 minutes.**

   This process releases saffron's flavor and color to the fullest!

3. **Add the liquid (and the crushed threads, unless you want to go to the trouble to try to remove them) to the dish.**

Thyme

It's about time you learned about thyme! A symbol of courage in the ancient cultures of the Mediterranean, this herb not only packs a strong aromatic flavor but also has antimicrobial properties that protect you from infection. Thyme, either fresh or dried, is a rich source of minerals, such as potassium, which helps control blood pressure, and iron, which is key for red blood cell formation.

Add a whole sprig of fresh thyme when you're roasting vegetables, chicken, or fish (but because of its tough stems, remove the sprig before consuming). Alternatively, add a pinch of dried thyme when cooking up meat or eggs for a ton of flavor in a small amount.

Chapter 18

Ten Studies on or Related to the Mediterranean Diet

. . . .

In This Chapter

▶ Looking at studies from around the world

▶ Seeing the benefit of key ingredients of the Mediterranean diet

▶ Highlighting key findings about disease prevention or mitigation

. . . .

*I*nterest in the relationship between the Mediterranean region and the
longevity of its denizens was sparked in middle of the 20th century when
folks began to notice that people in southern Europe seemed to be living
longer than people who lived in northern Europe and the United States. Since
then, several studies have been conducted trying to find the reason. Here are
ten of them.

The Seven Countries Study

Funded by a grant from the National Heart Institute and lead by Ancel Keys,
this decades-long study, which began in the 1950s, was one of the first
to examine the link between lifestyle and disease. Specifically, the Seven
Countries study followed population of men, ages 40 to 59, from seven countries (Finland, Greece, Italy, Japan, the Netherlands, the U.S., and Yugoslavia),
looking for association among diet, known risk factors, and the prevalence of
heart attacks and stroke.

The study's major findings include the observation that the risk of heart
attack and stroke is directly related to the level of total serum cholesterol, a
finding that held true for all groups studied, and that having high cholesterol
and being overweight or obese was associated with increased cancer deaths.

Although it didn't specifically study the Mediterranean diet, researchers observed that southern Europe had far fewer coronary deaths than northern Europe and the United States did, even when factoring in other known risks like age, smoking, blood pressure, and physical activity. This observation drew attention to diet as a key health factor and was supported by the fact that, as the people in the Mediterranean region began to shift from active lifestyles and healthy eating patterns to the less-active lifestyles and Western-influenced diets, the incidences of heart disease also increased.

This study is still important today because more people in the Mediterranean regions studied no longer eat in their traditional way, and those regions show higher occurrences of heart disease.

The SUN Project

The SUN Project, from the University of Navarro, Spain, was an ongoing study that sought to identify dietary causes of various health conditions, such as high blood pressure, diabetes, obesity, and heart disease. The study involved thousands of participants whom researchers followed up with and assessed every two years between 1999 and 2010. This project produced some interesting findings:

- Participants who followed a Mediterranean-style diet were less likely to develop type 2 diabetes. Even those who had high risk factors for type 2 diabetes (including older age, family history of diabetes, and a history of smoking) but followed the diet pattern strictly had an 83 percent relative reduction for developing the disease.

- Participants who ate a diet rich in olive oil had a reduced risk of hypertension (a finding that was statistically significant only among the men) and heart disease.

- Those whose diets included trans-unsaturated fatty acids were at greater risk of depression, while a weak inverse association was found between depression risk and monounsaturated fatty acids, polyunsaturated fatty acids, and olive oil (that is, the greater the consumption of healthy fats, the lower the risk for depression).

The PREDIMED Trial

The PREDIMED (*Prevención con Dieta Mediterránea*) trial, conducted in Spain and launched in 2003 with results published in 2013, was designed to determine whether, and to what degree, a Mediterranean diet prevents cardiovascular disease. It specifically compared a low-fat diet to a Mediterranean diet, supplemented with either extra-virgin olive oil or tree nuts, to see which was most effective at preventing heart disease, heart attacks, and strokes. The randomly selected participants who were at high risk for heart disease were divided into three groups:

✔ Those who followed a Mediterranean diet supplemented with tree nuts, which are high in polyphenols, monounsaturated fat, and polyunsaturated fat.

✔ Those who followed a Mediterranean diet supplemented with extra-virgin olive oil, which is rich in polyphenols and monounsaturated fat.

✔ Those who were instructed to lower their dietary fat intake.

As analysis of the groups progressed, the decision was made to end the trial early because ample evidence, in even a relatively short amount of time, showed that a Mediterranean-based diet, whether supplemented with nuts or extra-virgin olive oil, reduced the risk of heart disease by a whopping 30 percent.

The EPIC Project

The goal of the EPIC (European Prospective Investigation into Cancer) project was to explore the relationship between diet, lifestyle, and cancer, as well as other chronic diseases, like heart disease. It was the largest study of diet and health ever, involving over half a million people (most between the ages of 35 and 70 years old) across ten European countries: Denmark, France, Germany, Greece, Italy, the Netherlands, Norway, Spain, Sweden, and the United Kingdom.

Here are the key findings:

✔ You can lower your risk of high blood pressure by consuming less salt and more potassium.

✔ Diets high in fiber seem to offer protection against colorectal cancer risk, while diets high in red and processed meats increase the risk. Other factors that increase colorectal cancer risk include obesity and low physical activity.

✔ Being overweight or obese increases the risk for several types of cancer.

✔ Being overweight, being physically inactive, and consuming a high-fat diet increase breast cancer risk.

✔ High blood glucose levels increase the risk of heart disease.

Bottom line: You can add years to your life by engaging in these key behaviors: being physically active, eating at least five servings of fruits and vegetables a day (the Mediterranean diet has you eating between seven and ten servings), moderating how much alcohol you drink, and not smoking.

Research from the University of Louisiana's College of Pharmacology

A healthy brain has 100 billion nerve cells (neurons) that connect in an intricate web, called a *neuron forest*. Signals that form memories, ideas, and feelings travel from neuron to neuron in this forest. In a brain afflicted with Alzheimer's, problems occur when the two key proteins stop functioning properly and result in plaques and tangles being formed:

- Plaques form when *beta-amyloid* (sticky pieces of larger proteins) cluster together.
- Tangles form when the *tau protein,* whose job is to keep information flowing smoothly along the neuron highway, begins to collapse and twist on itself.

At this point, the cells, deprived of nutrients, die.

In the study, researchers showed that *oleocanthal,* a compound in extra virgin olive oil, helps decrease the accumulation of beta-amyloid in the brain by enhancing the production of other proteins and enzymes thought to be critical in removing beta-amyloid. The implication was that following a Mediterranean diet that features extra virgin olive oil has the potential to reduce the risk of Alzheimer's and other dementias.

Here's what's particularly interesting about his study: Previously people assumed that the protective agent in extra virgin olive oil was its healthy monounsaturated fats. Now researchers are taking a closer look a the protective qualities of oleocanthal.

The NIH-AARP Diet and Health Study

Together the National Institutes of Health and AARP (formerly known as the American Association of Retired Persons) conducted a study that investigated the link between diet and health. Seeking to gather information on lifestyle and diet for over half a million people, the AARP mailed over 3 million questionnaires in 1995 and 1996 to members 50 to 71 years old in California; Florida; Pennsylvania; New Jersey; North Carolina; Louisiana; Atlanta, Georgia; and Detroit, Michigan. More than half a million people responded, making this one of the largest studies of diet and health. In 2004, the organization conducted a follow-up survey.

The NIH-AARP Diet and Health study published in the *Archives of Internal Medicine* in 2007 found that people who closely adhered to a Mediterranean-style diet were 12 to 20 percent less likely to die from cancer and all causes.

The ATTICA Study

The ATTICA study, published in the September 2005 issue of the *American Journal of Clinical Nutrition,* measured the total antioxidant capacity of men and women in Greece. It found that the participants who followed a traditional Mediterranean diet had an 11 percent higher antioxidant capacity than those who didn't adhere to a traditional diet. The findings also showed that the participants who followed the traditional diet the most had 19 percent lower oxidized LDL (bad) cholesterol concentrations, which may potentially lower the risk of developing heart disease.

Harvard School of Public Health Study

Beginning in 1976, researchers from the Harvard School of Public Health followed 88,000 healthy women and found that the risk of colon cancer was 2.5 times higher in women who ate beef, pork, or lamb daily compared with those who ate those meats once a month or less. They also found that the risk of getting colon cancer was directly correlated to the amount of meat eaten.

2008 Study Reviews Regarding Cancer Risk

In addition to ingredient-specific studies, the diet as a whole has some promising research. A 2008 study review published in the *British Medical Journal* showed that following a traditional Mediterranean diet reduced the risk of dying from cancer by 9 percent.

That same year, the *American Journal of Clinical Nutrition* published a study that showed that, among post menopausal women, those who followed a traditional Mediterranean diet were 22 percent less likely to develop breast cancer. Although more research is needed in this area, you can enjoy a Mediterranean diet and know that you're helping improve your odds against cancer.

A study of 26,000 Greek people published in the *British Journal of Cancer* showed that using more olive oil cut cancer risk by 9 percent.

Study from Second University of Naples

A 2009 study from the Second University of Naples in Italy, published in the *Annals of Internal Medicine*, found that diabetics who followed a Mediterranean diet instead of a low-fat diet had better glycemic control and were less likely to need diabetes medication.

Chapter 19

Ten Easy but Effective Ways to Give Your Life a Mediterranean Boost

. . . .

In This Chapter

▶ Changing your portions sizes and the way you arrange your plate

▶ Focusing on healthy fats and whole foods

▶ Incorporating more fruits and vegetables into your diet

. . . .

*E*ven if you're not ready to commit full-time to the Mediterranean diet, you can still reap health benefits by making small changes. The following sections offer ten easy suggestions that will give your diet and your life a Mediterranean boost.

Snuggle Up to Olive Oil

Studies show that olive oil, specifically extra-virgin olive oil, helps lowers your risk of a variety of ailments, including cancer, Alzheimer's disease, and hypertension, in addition to providing other benefits.

Therefore, one of the best things you can do for your health is to begin using olive oil in place of other fat sources. Chapter 8 goes into detail on the health benefits of olive oil and the different kinds of olive oils you can choose from.

Reapportion Your Plate

Unlike the typical meals you're probably used to, in which meat (usually red) and a starch (usually some sort of potato) take up most, if not all, of the plate, a plate in a Mediterranean meal is apportioned differently: half, if not more, is devoted to fruits and vegetables, another quarter to the starch (usually a whole grain), and the last quarter to a protein source (usually seafood or lean meat). Even if you don't change what you're eating, you can make a huge, healthy difference simply by making your plate look more like one you'd find at a Mediterranean table.

Reduce Portion Sizes

Along with changing the way you apportion the different food groups (as explained in the preceding section), you can also make your diet more healthy just by paying attention to portion sizes. Pay particular attention to the less healthy things on your plate, like meat.

Cereal bowls are now the size of serving bowls, and dinner plates may as well be platters. So a great — and easy — way to reduce portion sizes without giving it too much thought is to simply use smaller dishes. Dust off your salad plates and condiment bowls. Believe it or not, the recommended portion sizes fit rather neatly on the smaller dishes.

Opt for Whole Grains over Refined

Whenever you're eating grain — bread, rice, cereal, and so on — go for the whole grain variety. Instead of white rice, choose brown. Instead of processed cereal, try oatmeal. And nowadays, with all the whole-grain bread options, you can get just about any kind of bread — pita, hamburger bun, hoagie roll, tortilla, dinner roll, and so on — in a whole grain variety. They're healthier, fill you up faster, and keep you full longer. Go to Chapter 11 for more information.

Keep Fruit and Veggies Handy

Seven to ten serving of fruits and vegetables a day — that's what the Mediterranean diet calls for. Even if you're completely committed to the diet, you may struggle to fit in this many servings, especially if your diet heretofore included, maybe, one or two servings — on a good day. An easy way to boost your consumption of the fruit and veggie group is to make sure you have fresh fruit and vegetables (carrots, sweet peppers, and so on) handy and ready to eat.

Chapter 10 lists several varieties of fruits and vegetables that are common in the Mediterranean and explains the nutrients and health benefits they offer.

Toss Nuts into Everything

Okay, not everything. After all, these nutritious nuggets are calorie-dense, which means it's easy to over indulge and get more calories than you need. But you can reap the benefits of nuts by including them as part of your meal plan: Sprinkle them on salads. Add them to oatmeal with a sprinkle of cinnamon. Enjoy a tablespoon of nut butter (peanut butter, almond butter, or cashew butter, for example) with fresh fruit.

Chapter 9 has the details on serving sizes and a variety of suggestions to help you incorporate nuts and seeds into your diet.

Commit to Eating Seafood at Least Twice a Week

Coastal living in the Mediterranean brings a rich variety of delicious, fresh seafood, and you see no shortage of fish and shellfish entrees and sides in the Mediterranean diet. If you're don't generally eat seafood, or if the seafood you eat is generally breaded and fried, have we got a treat for you.

Although fatty fish, like salmon, offers some of the biggest health benefits, any fish or seafood is a good choice. Preparing it can be a piece of cake, too: Simply brush it with olive oil, season it with a little salt and pepper, and bake it for a quick, easy meal.

Head to Chapter 12 for guidelines and more information.

Move Your Bones

The Mediterranean diet is about more than food. It's also about living life to its fullest: You don't have to join a gym, invest in exercise equipment, or devote all your free time to crunches and squats. You just have to get up and get moving! Take a walk. Garden. Help your kid learn to roller skate. Even cleaning house counts.

Laugh, Deeply, Once a Day

Laughter doesn't get the attention it deserves. But studies have demonstrated that smiling — even fake smiling — can lift a mood. So imagine what a good laugh can do. In fact, the saying that laugher is the best medicine has some truth to it. A 1989 study testing the effects of laughter found the following

- ✔ Laughter decreased the amount of cortisol (a hormone released under stress) in the blood more quickly for the laughing subjects than those in the control group.
- ✔ Laughter increased the number of immune cells that attack viruses.

Laughter also gives your body a workout. Researchers at the University of Michigan calculated that 20 minutes of laughter was as good for the lungs as 3 minutes on a rowing machine. So find something to laugh about, and as you're laughing, think of all the good you're doing your body.

Eat Your Veggies First

Regardless of how you apportion the food groups on your plate — whether the bulk goes to vegetables or fruits, as the Mediterranean diet promotes, or your vegetable is still a little dish off the side, as is typical of Western diet — eat the vegetable first. If you're someone who loves your veggies, this strategy lets you indulge in a favorite right off the bat, and if you're not a big fan of vegetables, it ensure that you get all the nutrients vegetables have to offer before you fill up with the other things on your plate. And in either case, by first tucking into the vegetables — which are generally the lower calorie items on your plate — you just may find that you have less room for the higher calorie items, like the meat and starch.

Include a Fruit or Veggie at Every Meal and Snack

Many folks who are accustomed to the traditional Western diet may struggle to fit in the seven to ten servings of fruits and vegetables a day. One way to make the goal easier is to include a fruit or veggie serving at every meal and in every snack. And because the serving sizes are probably smaller than you think (refer to Chapter 10), you'll fill your quota easily. A main dish salad, for example, can easily make up two servings, and a handful of raisins another serving.

Metric Conversion Guide

*N*ote: The recipes in this book weren't developed or tested using metric measurements. There may be some variation in quality when converting to metric units.

Common Abbreviations

Abbreviation(s)	What It Stands For
cm	Centimeter
C., c.	Cup
G, g	Gram
kg	Kilogram
L, l	Liter
lb.	Pound
mL, ml	Milliliter
oz.	Ounce
pt.	Pint
t., tsp.	Teaspoon
T., Tb., Tbsp.	Tablespoon

Volume

U.S. Units	Canadian Metric	Australian Metric
¼ teaspoon	1 milliliter	1 milliliter
½ teaspoon	2 milliliters	2 milliliters
1 teaspoon	5 milliliters	5 milliliters
1 tablespoon	15 milliliters	20 milliliters
¼ cup	50 milliliters	60 milliliters
⅓ cup	75 milliliters	80 milliliters
½ cup	125 milliliters	125 milliliters
⅔ cup	150 milliliters	170 milliliters
¾ cup	175 milliliters	190 milliliters
1 cup	250 milliliters	250 milliliters
1 quart	1 liter	1 liter
1½ quarts	1.5 liters	1.5 liters
2 quarts	2 liters	2 liters
2½ quarts	2.5 liters	2.5 liters
3 quarts	3 liters	3 liters
4 quarts (1 gallon)	4 liters	4 liters

Weight

U.S. Units	Canadian Metric	Australian Metric
1 ounce	30 grams	30 grams
2 ounces	55 grams	60 grams
3 ounces	85 grams	90 grams
4 ounces (¼ pound)	115 grams	125 grams
8 ounces (½ pound)	225 grams	225 grams
16 ounces (1 pound)	455 grams	500 grams (½ kilogram)

Length

Inches	Centimeters
0.5	1.5
1	2.5
2	5.0
3	7.5
4	10.0
5	12.5
6	15.0
7	17.5
8	20.5
9	23.0
10	25.5
11	28.0
12	30.5

Temperature (Degrees)

Fahrenheit	Celsius
32	0
212	100
250	120
275	140
300	150
325	160
350	180
375	190
400	200
425	220
450	230
475	240
500	260

Index

Author's Acknowledgments

I, Rachel, would like to say thank you to everyone at John Wiley & Sons for letting me be a part of this project on a topic I'm so passionate about. Thank you to Tracy Boggier for believing in me, yet again, and to Tracy Barr for her incredible work putting together a comprehensive book on all things Mediterranean. Also, thank you to my technical editor, Dr. Michael Lim, who ensured that the scientific info in this book is supported by the most current medical research.

This book could not have been completed without the amazing work of the health care professionals who authored the chapters on their specialty conditions: James Rippe, MD *(Heart Disease For Dummies);* John Marler, MD *(Stroke For Dummies);* Alan Rubin, MD *(Diabetes For Dummies);* Brent Agin, MD, and Sharon Perkins, RN *(Healthy Aging For Dummies);* and Alan P. Lyss, MD, Humberto M. Fagundes, MD, and Patricia Corrigan *(Chemotherapy & Radiation For Dummies).*

I'd like to give a huge shout-out to my fellow dietitians, Meri Raffetto, RD, and Wendy Jo Peterson, MS, RD, who authored *Mediterranean Diet Cookbook For Dummies* and contributed delicious recipes and information on the Mediterranean lifestyle to this title.

I'm forever grateful for my supportive family and friends, especially those who dine with me on Mediterranean fare (and put up with my babbling about food history and health benefits) and participate in aspects of this lifestyle with me (like being active and drinking wine!). Finally, thanks to you, the reader, for picking up this book to learn about the Mediterranean way. Opa!

Publisher's Acknowledgments

Senior Acquisitions Editor: Tracy Boggier

Editor: Tracy Barr

Technical Editor: Michael Lim, MD

Project Coordinator: Sheree Montgomery

Cover Image: ©iStockphoto.com/Kelly Cline